# CRITICAL CARE NURSING

# CRITICAL CARE NURSING

**Sanjeev Singh**

**ANMOL PUBLICATIONS PVT. LTD.**
**NEW DELHI - 110 002 (INDIA)**

**ANMOL PUBLICATIONS PVT. LTD.**
*H.O.:* 4374/4B, Ansari Road, Darya Ganj,
New Delhi-110 002 (India)
Ph.: 23278000, 23261597

*B.O.:* No. 1015, Ist Main Road, BSK IIIrd Stage
IIIrd Phase, IIIrd Block,
Bangalore - 560 085 (India)
Visit us at: www.anmolpublications.com

*Critical Care Nursing*



First Published, 2006



PRINTED IN INDIA

Printed at Mehra Offset Press, Delhi.

# Contents

# Preface

With an ability to think quickly, act decisively and stay calm when lives are at stake, critical-care nurses are among the in-demand healthcare professionals who make life-or-death decisions about patient care every day. Critical-care nurses treat patients at high risk for actual or potential life-threatening health problems and also tend to the emotional well being of those patients' families. That's no small task. Critical-care nurses draw on good communication skills, endless compassion and the ability to concentrate amid a patient crisis to succeed in their roles.

The aim of Critical Care Nursing is to provide critical care and acute care nurses with accurate, relevant, and useful information concerning the bedside care of critically and acutely ill patients. By reading this volume critical care and acute care nurses should benefit through increased knowledge concerning critical and acute care nursing practice, history of critical care, ethical issues and be able to use this knowledge to care for patients and their families in a more effective manner.

Comprehensive, logically organized, and easy to read, this text provides students with a solid base for their critical care nursing education. Encompassing history, procedures, skills and issues it offers thorough coverage, an emphasis on critical thinking, and a focus on care in critical care nursing. This volume addresses a number of key issues, including evidence-based practice, safety concerns, and end-of-life care.

The aim of this volume is to provide a concise repository of number of major concepts. In preparation of this book, the author has freely consulted large number of books and journals so no authenticity is claimed. Author is specially thankful to M/S Anmol Publications for shaping this book in its final form.

Suggestions for further improvement of this book are not only welcome but also greatly appreciated.

Author

# Chapter 1

# Critical Care Nursing

## INTRODUCTION

Critical care nursing is the nursing of people undergoing life-threatening physiological crises. According to the Association of Critical Care Nurses, "the scope of critical care nursing is defined by the dynamic interaction of the critically ill patient, the critical care nurse and the critical care environment". Critical care nursing may be distinguished from nursing practice in general by the severity of the patient's illness, the particular skills of the nurse, and the setting where the nursing is practiced. Joan Lynaugh and Julie Fairman distinguish two criteria inherent in the meaning of critical care. "First, the person receiving care is physiologically unstable and at risk of dying. Second, intensive care is usually given in the expectation or hope, however slim, of the person's survival. The relationship between them [these criteria] changes over time" Critical care units emerged in hospitals after World War II. Medical specialization, increasingly sophisticated medical technology, and advances in anesthesia, cardiology, and surgery influenced this phenomenon. Nathan Simon attributes the development of the modern intensive care unit (ICU) concept to three major forces. First, the recovery room experience in the 1940s and 1950s demonstrated to medicine and nursing the effectiveness of continuous nursing surveillance of very ill patients. Patients waking up after anesthesia and surgery could be monitored in one large room for immediate complications such as respiratory distress, cardiac or blood pressure abnormalities, or bleeding. Second, hospital planners proposed a progressive patient care concept: patients in hospitals would be grouped according to the amount and intensity of nursing care required. Their goal was efficiency – the best matching of nurses with patients. Third, complex technology, medical specialization, and new surgical procedures required more sophisticated postoperative nursing care. The development in the early 1960s of cardiopulmonary resuscitation (CPR) machines for monitoring heart rhythm (cardiac monitors) and DC (direct current) defibrillation for the treatment of lethal arrhythmias after heart attacks ushered in the era of the coronary care unit.

The Joint Commission on Accreditation of Healthcare Organizations defines a special care unit as one "that provides intensive care continuously on a 24-hour-a-day basis. Specific purpose special care units may include, but need not be limited to burn, cardiac, cardiovascular surgery, neonatal, respiratory units, and multipurpose special care units that usually include medical-surgical intensive care units or a combination of the above". The majority of all hospitals (61%) have one specific critical care unit providing combined medicalsurgical care. Medical centers or university teaching hospitals are likely to have more than one unit, each providing specialty care – for example, heart surgery, neurosurgery, organ transplant (liver, pancreas, kidney, heart, heart-lung, or bone marrow), pulmonary, or trauma units. Hence, intensive care is now a usual standard of care in hospitals. Patients may be admitted to an intensive care unit for an acute illness like pneumonia or a heart attack; for short-term management after specialized surgery such as coronary artery bypass surgery; or for long-term management of complications of either — for example, a patient on a ventilator for respiratory support after respiratory arrest during treatment for pneumonia.

The highly technical, highly specialized, patient care units that we now term "critical care units" have developed over the past 30 years. Today's ultra-modern intensive care unit is an outgrowth of a few units established prior to World War II for the care of postoperative patients who required close watching while awakening from general anesthesia. The polio epidemics of the 1950s spurred the realization that there are groups of patients with very acute illnesses who require a different, more intense kind of medical and nursing care than is generally available on the regular hospital wards, and that it is more efficient and effective to group these patients together. It became common to put such patients into recovery rooms, located next to operating room suites. The early trials with coronary care units confirmed the need for other specialized units, and "critical care" was off and running.

Any discussion of critical care today must include the major providers of continuous care—critical care nurses. Regardless of profession or specialty, all those involved in the care of critically in patients interact with ICU nurses. Learning about this group of care providers is useful in daily interactions and in the anlaysis of the many complex issues described in the other chapters of this book, such as decision making and resource allocation. The purpose of this chapter is to provide the reader with a brief review of the history and status of critical care nursing, as well as a description of the issues related to the role of the critical care nurse.

Critical care nurses represent a portion of the registered nurse population. A brief description of the entire population thus provides useful background information.

The nursing profession as a whole is composed predominantly of females (97%), with a median age of 38 years. Of those currently working, 70.8 percent are married;

46 percent are married and have children at home. Reflecting the dual roles required of working wives and mothers, 32 percent of employed nurses only work part-time. Two-thirds of all nurses were originally educated in hospital-based diploma programs. Seventeen percent graduated from a college or university-based Bachelor of Nursing program, and an additional 5 percent later returned to school to obtain their degree. Five percent of all nurses hold master's or doctoral degrees. Thirty-three percent of all admissions to basic nursing programs in 1979-80 were to B.Sc[N] programs. When compared to a 1970 survey, this study reflected increases in the number of registered nurses, the percent employed, the percent receiving a bachelor's degree as their initial educational preparation, and the percent of minority (including males) members. Decreases were shown in the average age and percent receiving their basic education in hospital-based programs.

Many of the challenges facing nurses today have their roots in these statistics. Nursing is a sex-segregated occupation. Unlike medicine, nursing loses a large number of its practitioners each year as women leave work to raise their families. In terms of educational preparation, nurses are a much more heterogeneous group than those in other health occupations; backgrounds of direct patient care providers range from a two-year community college education to a seven-year universitybased program for the clinical specialist. This makes it difficult, to say the least, for others to develop appropriate expectations of nurses, which often causes conflict. It seems unlikely that these characteristics will change rapidly, although the identified trends are expected to continue.

Regardless of the practice setting, all nurses share elements of a common philosophy. Most of the significant contributions and conflicts of ICU nurses stem from this philosophical base.

The cornerstone of the nursing philosophy is caring, the raison d'être of the nurse. The word "nurse" stems from the Latin word for nurture; this origin provides us with the nurse's first obligation—to the patient—and is the source of one of the most persistent metaphors for nurse—that is, a mother substitute. , This image exists in the minds of the public and many other care providers, who expect the nurse/mother to embody all the positive characteristics associated with motherhood: caring, gentleness, and devotion. It also underlies many of the conflicts as others, particularly physicians and even some nurse administrators, expect subservience and acquiescence.

Kalisch and Kalisch conducted an exhaustive study of public media and confirmed the predominance of this image of the nurse in television and literature. , They found three basic portrayals: nurse as man's companion, man's destroyer, and man's mother or mother of his children. A content analysis of the personal attributes of nurses on television revealed that nurses rated high on obedience, permissiveness, and conformity; physicians scored high on sophistication, intelligence, rationality, and aggression. It was not until the 1960s that the media gained some recognition of nurses as real persons, with both positive and negative traits, who have some professional identity and assume responsibility for their own actions. Unfortunately, the 1970s brought a return to the use of nurse characters as sexual mascots for men, particularly physicians—stereotypes which were disparaging to both groups.

The abundance of definitions of nursing in the nursing literature is an indication of the degree to which this profession or occupation is in transition. All definitions, however, appear to have common elements. First is the notion of assisting, helping, ministering, or providing care; all of these actions are differentiated from curing or providing a specific technologic service. Thus, the basis of nursing activities is quite general and broad, and is not confined to a particular act or technique.

Next, all definitions refer to the recipients of care in an equally broad fashion: individuals, groups, families, peers—

in fact, anyone who is experiencing a "broad range of health-illness phenomena." There is generally a specific absence of reference to patients as sufferers of disease or seekers of certain services.

The last element, appearing more often in recent definitions, refers to the methodology used by the nurse to assist individuals, a specific art and science of nursing. This idea is in direct contrast to the "mother" image and notions of nursing as a natural female function. It is perhaps in critical care nursing that the nurse's goal of "caring for" is most obviously dependent upon the utilization of technical skills and basic science concepts. The Association of Critical-Care Nurses further defines critical care nursing as "the utilization of the nursing process (assessment, planning, implementation, and evaluation) in the prevention of or intervention in life-threatening situations." At its most fundamental level, then, it can be said that all of nursing has a care, rather than cure, orientation, a wellness (prevention of disease or crisis)—in addition to illness—concern, and a whole person—rather than organ or subsystem—focus.

Further analysis of the philosophy of nursing must include reference to the nurse's role in the health care society, the source of the nurse's accountability. The hospital nurse today leads a somewhat schizophrenic existence. The institutional bureaucracy expects the allegiance of the nurse as an employee, the physician expects the loyalty of his handmaiden, and the nurse expects him/herself to be accountable to the patient. Each of these allegiances bears further discussion.

As an employee, the nurse certainly has contractual obligations to the hospital. This employee status is problematic in two regards. The hospital, like all organizations, imposes certain rules that reflect institutional values, such as growth, stability, and risk minimization. These rules, however, may be in direct conflict with the nurse's perceptions of his/her obligations to the patient. Providing access to medical records or information about the patient's hospitalization is a common example of an activity that might present such a conflict. In addition to the dilemmas posed by the conflicts themselves, this state of divided loyalties encourages nurses to substitute hospital policies for action guides developed from individual reasoning. Consequently, "policy" is frequently cited as a reason for doing or not doing something.

Loyalty to the physician has long been considered one of the most essential qualities of the "good nurse," and is probably one of the most persistently disturbing issues to nurses today. The extent to which the nurse perceives an obligation, and the exact nature of that obligation, vary considerably with the nurse's education, experience, and practice location. It is an element of philosophy that has undergone tremendous change over the years.

Unquestionably, the history of medicine and nursing reflects the origins of the nurse's role as a handmaiden who is under the control and guidance of the physician, has neither the ability nor the need to act independently, and owes allegiance to her master. Contrast this with the obligations of today's nurse set forth in the Nurses Association Code for Nurses:

> The nurse acts to safeguard the client and the public when health care and safety are affected by the incompetent, unethical, or illegal practice of any person.
>
> The nurse assumes responsibility and accountability for individual nursing judgments and actions.

The interpretive statements published with the Code further emphasize the nurse's first and foremost responsibility—to the patient, not to the physician, with whom the nurse works in a collaborative, not dependent, fashion. The activities of the nurse are considered a primary and separate patient service. Although this service is obviously related to the work of the physician, the nurse is not considered only in the context of a physician's aide.

It may be argued that we have all come a long way from these historical origins. Yet, the existence of day-to-day conflict, reflected in numerous analyses in the literature and actual court litigation, speaks otherwise. As recently as 1977, a physician's complaint resulted in a nurse's license being revoked by the State Board of Nursing for "unprofessional conduct." At the patient's request, the nurse had provided the patient with objective information about alternatives to the cancer therapy recommended by the physician.

Obviously, the philosophical ideals expressed here are not shared by all nurses. However, they are ideals and concepts to which all nurses are exposed in their education and socialization. As such, they may serve as background for a further examination of the critical care nursing role.

## STATUS OF CRITICAL CARE NURSING

The development of critical care nursing was a natural corollary to the growth of critical care units. The first specialty organization, like the first specialty units, was of coronary care nurses. As critical care broadened to include the care of patients who did not have cardiac diseases, the Association of Coronary Care Nurses expanded to become the Association of Critical Care Nurses. By 1979, membership had grown from several hundred to over 39,000.

More significant than the numerical growth of critical care nurses was the development of the science of critical care nursing. In 1975, the recognition of the need for a defined core body of knowledge resulted in the publication of the first *Core Curriculum for Critical Care Nursing*. The development of the certification exam occurred several years later. Today's critical care nurse considers him/herself a professional and a specialist.

As the numbers of critical care nurses have grown, increasing attention has been paid to the specialization of this branch of nursing. A particular focus has been comparisons between ICU and non-ICU nurses. As stated by Hay and Oken, the rationale is: "It stands to reason that nurses who operate special machines and perform special procedures for special patients must be special too!"

Most surveys describe ICU nurses as younger than other nurses, with a slightly higher percent having a B.S.N. degree. - Grout's study of 1,238 ICU nurses revealed that the major reasons for choosing ICU nursing were the opportunity for learning, the intellectual challenge, and the opportunity to develop proficiency in nursing skills. Although research has focused on the qualities or personality traits that differentiate ICU nurses from others, results have been equivocal.

In one of the earliest studies, Gentry found that ICU nurses reported more depression, hostility, and anxiety than non-ICU nurses. He identified situational stresses of the work environment of the critical care unit as significant variables. On the other hand, Dear's study of 100 nurses found critical care nurses to be more highly satisfied with their work, with no differences in the level of perceived autonomy, locus of control, or turnover rates. Looking specifically at stress tolerance, Maloney and Bartz reported that critical care nurses scored higher in alienation and external control, and were more likely to seek challenge. However, another study by Maloney demonstrated that non-ICU nurses scored significantly higher than ICU nurses in both state and trait anxiety, job dissatisfaction, and reporting of personal and family problems. Benton and White examined data on 565 nurses of various specialties (ICU, obstetrics, medicine, surgery, and pediatrics) and found that patient care itself was the job factor most important to satisfaction, followed by having an adequate number of personnel per shift; pay differential for experience, written job descriptions, and promotional opportunities were least important. The ICU group's rankings for these factors were the same as those of the total group.

As outlined above, many of the comparisons of critical care nurses and other nurses have concentrated on measuring the stress to which the ICU nurse is subjected, the reactions of the nurse to stress, or the personality traits and defenses needed to cope with stress. This reflects a general perception of ICUs as stressful environments and a persistent, unsupported conviction that there must be some differences, some unique characteristics, that attract nurses to the ICU. This view has been encouraged by the recognition of the "burnout" phenomenon-that is, the disillusionment and emotional exhaustion associated with human service occupations which comes of personal surrender to overwhelming demands and external, unchanging realities.

In his review of stress and intensive care nursing, Friedman cautions that the environmental demands that are perceived by one nurse as a "stressor" may represent a "satisfier" to another. Nevertheless, certain factors do reappear in the literature as common or frequently reported stressors: conflict with other health care providers; inadequate staffing patterns; unresponsive nursing leadership; lack of recognition by physicians; lack of support in dealing with death and dying; dealing with families.

Eisendrath points out the likelihood of conflict arising from the similarities between many ICUs and family systems, in which the medical director is "father," head nurse is "mother," and the nursing and house staffs are "children." This idea is consistent with the historical roots of the nurse-physician relationship. While it could provide an emotionally supportive base for young practitioners of both disciplines, it also leads to "sibling rivalry" and a repression of the growth of the "children."

In addition to recognizing that individuals vary in their perceptions and identifications of stressors, it should be noted that there may be significant differences among the various types of intensive care units. These differences may account for widely varying perceptions of stress and/or job satisfaction. For example, surgical intensive care units typically have a younger patient population with a shorter length of stay. The patients most often present with one or two major problems. The focus of care is to resolve or monitor those problems for a brief, defined, high-risk period of time. The frequent arrival of patients directly from the operating room provides a population that is most unstable and dependent upon caregivers for life-sustaining measures. Medical intensive care unit patients, on the other hand, tend to be older, have a higher mortality rate, and present with chronic diseases and multisystem problems requiring the use of more consultants. Variation among patients is great, ranging from the brief, one-day monitoring required by overdose patients to the prolonged, highly complex care required by septic, bone marrow transplant patients. Coronary care units have a patient population that is generally awake and alert, many of whom are experiencing their first major illness. While the focus of their care is on only one organ system, it requires in-depth investigation and intervention. The restful, quiet environment of the coronary unit provides a vivid contrast to the highly technologic focus of medical and surgical units.

The significance of these differences lies in the match between the individual nurse and the challenges and satisfiers presented by the particular environment. For example, the nurse who gains the greatest degree of satisfaction and reward from working overtime with patients and families, designing comprehensive care plans, and having the opportunity to see the fruition of his or her plans over weeks or months is likely to be dissatisfied with the environment of a surgical unit, and will find the constant, rapid turnover of patients stressful. The nurse who enjoys the short-term, highly defined, and intense relationships typical of the SICU, where priorities of care are well established, may perceive the slow progress of the MICU patient as a stressor.

Strategies proposed to deal with these stressors and prevent burnout primarily focus on interpersonal techniques, such as talking with others, group meetings, and role-playing sessions. Cook and Madrino's work on perceived stress and situational supports confirms the importance of these interpersonal factors. In their study, the highest correlation with perceived situational support was positive coworker relationships. After administering a Stress Audit to 1,800 nurses, Bailey, Steffen, and Grout also found that interpersonal staff relationships were among the three most important satisfiers.

## The Critical Care Team

The concept of multidisciplinary teams gained popularity in the 1970s. The increased complexity of illnesses and therapies required by critically ill patients mandated that planning, provision, and evaluation of care be extended beyond the primary doctor and nurse. Clinical pharmacists, dieticians, respiratory therapists, psychologists, social workers, and many others have become regular participants in critical care teams. In fact, most texts addressing management and organization of contemporary critical care units mention the need to have a team.

According to Adler and Shoemaker, in AACN's text on management, physicians and nurses originally formed teams in order to overcome political obstacles to the growth and development of intensive care units, and provide the support system necessary for the unit personnel. Meltzer, one of the earliest proponents of coronary care units, called the team approach "the most distinguishing characteristic of the coronary care concept," referring to the improved communication, efficiency, and organization that resulted from this structure. This concept has also gained popularity abroad. In describing England's "intensive therapy units," Ledingham also addresses the need for multidisciplinary activities and the regular involvement of ancillary staff, physiotherapists, and technicians necessitated by the diverse range of equipment used. The National Institute of Health, in a Consensus Development Conference in 1983, defined critical care as "a multidisciplinary and multiprofessional medical/nursing field . . ."

The question of whether this multidisciplinary group is truly a team has been addressed by Erde. He points out that teams are generally understood to be democracies, yet the health care "team" rarely elects their leader. In addition to the physician's being self-appointed, patients expect him to be the captain. Also, women lack men's socialization to team behavior and are poorly prepared to operate as equal team members.

Erde begins his discussion with a definition of the term *team*, which includes the proviso that members share a common goal and a common set of norms. This definition in itself raises questions about the degree to which the health care team's goals and beliefs are truly the same. For example, the list below presents four beliefs held by many critical care nurses:

1. The nurse is an independent professional.
2. Care may be more important than cure.
3. The quality of life may be the most important outcome.
4. The nurse's primary responsibility is to the patient; all nursing actions must, therefore, be guided by the nurse's judgment of what is in the patient's best interest.

These are certainly basic rules, or norms, applicable to the practice of the critical care team; however, the extent to which these norms are recognized and accepted by all team members (even all nurses) is doubtful.

Contrary to the team notion, We believe critical care today is provided by a multidisciplinary group that interacts in a relatively undefined network of relationships, and has some degree of cohesiveness and identity. This cohesiveness is the product of the group's shared commitment to patient welfare, which members may or may not define in the same manner. The group identity is a function of both the shared commitment and the structure afforded by the organizational arrangement of duties, such as ICU medical director, head nurse, staff nurse, ICU social worker, and so on.

The formal organizational structure, informal distribution of work, and expectations of coworkers vary considerably from setting to setting. Major differences in norms may be observed by comparing the large specialty units found in major teaching hospitals with the small, mixed medical-surgical units of smaller community hospitals. Large, complex organizations typically have a wider variety of workers, each with a highly defined specialty. Since each member of the work group becomes quite expert in a narrow area, there is little overlapping of roles. Territorial concerns and tensions are not uncommon, as each member of the group struggles to protect his "turf." In contrast, the nurse working in a small hospital usually performs a multitude of roles and must be a generalist, equally skilled in caring for medical, surgical, coronary, and perhaps pediatric patients. While the nurse in some units has 24-hour access to IV, respiratory and physical therapists, laboratory and EKG technicians, transporters, and clerks, the community hospital nurse may have to assume all of these roles at different times.

The presence of house staff (residents, interns, and medical students) is also a significant variable in the development of group norms. Nurses who are accustomed to working with young student physicians, rather than primarily with older, senior, experienced physicians, are far more likely to adopt a questioning attitude and view physicians as less than omniscient. It is a curious paradox that nurses who work in a small community hospital ICU are often very independent because there is no physician present in the hospital during evening and night hours; yet, they are more likely to view the physician as the ultimate authority over all aspects of patient care, including nursing care.

There are several other characteristic differences between small community ICUs and those in medical centers that may be relevant to this discussion. As mentioned earlier, the relatively recent changes in nursing philosophy that advocate a more autonomous role for the nurse, with less emphasis on responsibility and accountability to the physician, are becoming more popular. It is the younger practitioners who are more likely to question and refute the norms of previous generations. The majority of new graduates seek employment in larger hospitals, particularly those affiliated with a university, because of the perceived challenges and learning opportunities. Thus, the nurses who are most likely to strongly reject the old norms and demand recognition for equal professional status are concentrated in the larger hospitals.

The nursing leadership provided in academic settings also supports the questioning of traditional relationships and role restructuring. As one would expect, the highest percentage of nurses with advanced academic preparation (master's and doctoral degrees) is found in university settings. These are the individuals who are the strongest proponents of the professionalization of nursing. The influence of their leadership and the organizational power of some nursing departments should not be underestimated. The young, inexperienced practitioner who is employed in this setting is exposed to a very different environment and very different role models.

In contrast, the ICU nurse who chooses a small town hospital often has limited access to professional nursing resources. He/she becomes a member of a work group that is older, more stable, and has traditional norms and values. As one nurse phrased it, "The physicians are our biggest resource. When we live, work, and socialize together in a small community, our relationship goes beyond the few minutes of professional contact in the ICU."

The last variable that influences the operation of the "team" and the specific roles of members is the hierarchy within each specific unit. Units with consistent individuals in designated positions of leadership are more likely to form a stable team. The two most pivotal positions are those of physician director and head nurse. If there is no physician director, the physician-in-charge changes every month, or the physician director is not actively involved with the care of all patients on a daily basis, staff members are not likely to develop the kind of cohesive team described in the literature. The same is true of units in which the head nurse position is either vacant or filled by a nurse who does not accept the team concept.

These considerations are obviously generalizations, and many exceptions may be found. They are also not to be construed as determinants of the quality of care provided in any setting. Rather, they are intended to provide a description of some of the organizational factors that influence the critical care nurse's role and role relationships.

This variation in the nurse's role is evident in the specific tasks for which he/she is responsible and the nature of the nurse-patient relationship. Obviously, the nurse is responsible for providing what is generally accepted as "nursing care"—for example, monitoring patient status, administering treatments and medications, changing dressings, personal hygiene, discharge teaching, and so on. However, this description of tasks is not necessarily a full description of the nurse's role.

Aside from the educational preparation necessary to assume the tasks mentioned, there are other characteristics of the nursing role that enable the critical care nurse to perform a broader function. The two roles which have received the greatest attention are those of coordinator and advocate.

Developments in modern hospitals have created conditions in the intensive care unit that are conducive to having nurses assume different roles. The extensive increases in the amount and complexity of technology have left the consumer feeling that he is indeed a stranger in a strange land, ill-equipped to deal with this foreign environment. Advances in the breadth and depth of knowledge in the natural sciences have spurred an increase in specialization, thus increasing the fragmentation of care. Each organ and each disease entity is now managed by its own physician or paramedic, with no one looking after the owner. While the consumer movement of the 1980s is perhaps overdue, it has further widened the gap between the public's expectations and the ability of any one caregiver to meet an of the patient's biological, social, and emotional needs.

This gap has given rise to the notion that patients require someone to coordinate their care. Corless describes the coordinator's responsibilities as "ensuring that there are no gaps in care and that the patient receives the therapies which are required for his or her wellbeing." Speaking of the need to restructure roles, Aiken describes the "continuing synthesis of the prescriptions of many physicians and professional surveillance of multiple diagnostic and treatment regimes."34 In general, the coordinator is viewed as one who can put the pieces together, ensure continuity and thoroughness of care, and establish the priorities of care.A closely related role is that of the advocate, a person who can assist the patient in exercising his or her rights. Annas specified four activities of the patient rights advocate:

1. Guaranteeing that the patient has access to all medical records;
2. Monitoring the quality of care;
3. Gaining access to services or consultants;
4. Participating in all discussions relating to patient care as the patient's representative.

Other functions might include that of ombudsman—that is, someone to whom the patient can turn with questions or concerns, and lay counselor—that is, someone to assist the patient in evaluating decisions and resolving conflicts.

Those who believe the nurse should assume these roles point to the unique features of the nurse's educational preparation and relationship with the patient. As mentioned earlier, nurses are oriented towards caring for the whole person, rather than dealing with one subsystem. Their educational background prepares them for this focus. The Bachelor of Science in Nursing program educates generalists with equal preparation in the biological and social sciences. In addition, nurses are the only members of the health "team" who are continuous caregivers, present 24 hours a day. All other care – medical care, spiritual guidance, social service support, physical therapy – is episodic and transient; nursing care is provided from the first moment of hospitalization to the last. The recent growth of primary nursing, in which one nurse is expected to plan, direct, and evaluate all nursing care, has made the notion of the nurse as coordinator even more attractive.

Another characteristic that makes the nurse even more suitable for the coordinator and advocate roles is the peer relationship that is possible between nurse and patient. It is ironic that it is the public image of the nurse as a mother who performs a natural function in a warm and caring fashion – an image decried by nurses struggling to achieve recognition and professional status as scientists – that enables nurses to avoid what may be a crisis of alienation in medicine. Bergen, Lindenthal, and Thomas describe two current opinions about physicians. At worst, they are villains in a "drama of good guys vs. bad guys." At best, they are technicians who neglect the total patient and his psychological needs as a result of their necessary preoccupation with the biological realities of disease. The patient's alienation from the physician is intensified by a "rule of silence" imposed on patients, who avoid confronting physicians and sharing their hopes, wishes, and needs. ". . . [I]f we do not speak about our values that can give and withhold other's authority over us, it is because we forswear speaking in favor of the ancient dream that by our becoming an object for another, the other will surely deliver us from suffering." The patient expects no such deliverance from his nurse. Thus, he is free to unburden his worries and receive services which would never be demanded from the physician—for example, support, care coordination, and advocacy.

## Issues in critical care

As members of the largest group of caregivers, nurses perform an essential function in administering direct care to acutely ill patients. They are, by and large, a well-educated group with increasing preparation at the university and postgraduate levels. Their defined body of knowledge is applied in a unique fashion. In addition, their qualifications should enable them to fulfill both the coordinator and advocate roles. Why, then, are these roles not legitimized as belonging to the nurse. The ideas of nurse as coordinator and nurse as advocate are so attractive and supportable, that there must be very fundamental and pervasive reasons why these roles have yet to be actualized to any great extent.

The concepts of rights and duties may serve as the basis for an explanation. Veatch describes duties of station—that is, the specific duties that accrue when one assumes a role, such as coordinator or advocate—as a kind of promising; one promises to fulfill the expectations that are inherent in the role. In order for these duties to be legitimate, and for one to be obligated to fulfill the promise, one must have the *right* to fulfill the promise. Rights generally require the recognition or agreement of all parties involved. In this case, before the nurse can assume the duties of advocate or coordinator as part of the nursing role, other members of the health care establishment, such as physicians, hospital administrators, social workers, and so on, would have to accord to the nurse the right to be an advocate or coordinator. This is not done. Nurses—even critical care nurses—are generally accorded neither the autonomy nor the authority needed to enact these roles. Effectiveness in either role requires the ability to significantly affect the behavior and decisions of other care providers; this power, which is associated with professional status, has not yet been achieved by nurses.

Studies and descriptions of the reasons for the much-publicized nursing shortage of the late 1970s and early 1980s have repeatedly supported this description of the hospital hierarchy. The shortage was mostly attributable to the fact that the hospital has become a less satisfying place for nurses. This arises from: the absence of appropriate organizational and managerial arrangements between nurses, physicians, and hospitals that clearly recognize the appropriate role of nurses in modern medical practice. . . . There are fundamental incompatibilities in the present social contract between hospitals, physicians, and today's professional nurses. . . . Despite the fact that hospitalized patients are more acutely ill than ever before, there has been little recognition of the importance of the nurse's role in the new level of clinical decision making required by these very sick patients.

The Hospital Association prepared an issue paper and distributed it to hospital executives to assist in addressing the problem. They stated: "Hospitals need to provide autonomy for nurses, foster positive attitudes of physicians toward collaborative practice, and enhance availability and quality of support services. Frequent articles also appeared in the public media during this period. Most attributed the problem, as did a report in the *Wall Street Journal*, to the lack of respect from physicians, inadequate control over the content of nurses' work, poor working conditions, and inadequate pay for what nurses consider to be professional responsibility.

After studying the historical development of nursing, Levi identified functional redundancy as the key reason for nursing's failure to be recognized as a profession. She pointed out that all the jobs or tasks performed by nurses can also be performed by members of some other occupation.

For example, many hospitals utilize monitor technicians to observe and assess data and functioning of cardiac and hemodynamic monitors. In some settings, respiratory therapists assume responsibility for mechanical ventilators and care of patients' airways. Pharmacy technicians may distribute medications. Licensed practical nurses provide physical care in many smaller community hospital ICUS, in place of registered nurses. Registered nurses claim that they provide higher quality of care, and that this functional distribution adds to fragmentation of care. This view is obviously not shared by many others. The fact that nurses lack a monopoly over significant skills, such as physicians possess, makes it unlikely that society at large, and other health care providers in particular, will accord to nurses the power and prestige necessary to make advocacy or coordinating a viable role.

An extremely important issue in examining the nurse's role is the categorization of nursing as a sex-segregated occupation. In addition to its psychosociological and economic influences, this factor impacts upon nurses' struggles to achieve autonomy.

Ashley, one of nursing's most outspoken critics of the current social order, views misogyny, the hatred of women, as a destructively pervasive characteristic of virtually all of human existence. She discusses misogyny as an integral part of our society's patriarchal structure, and its effects on the health care culture. Describing the ancient origins of this patriarchy, she points to the genesis of woman as a secondary, derivative being who was the source of sin. Women's place in history has been reinforced as being weak, defective, and whole only when fulfilling the purpose of assisting or subjugating herself to man. The anti-female medical abuses criticized by feminists, such as the performing of unnecessary surgery and the excessive prescription of tranquilizers, are the inevitable result of an attitude that classifies women as sick by virtue of their sex. According to Ashley, these same misogynous myths are responsible for the fact that nurses have remained the servants of physicians. This is not seen as attributable to any aspect or characteristic of nurses or nursing; it is simply the result of its being an occupation in which women are the primary workers. In order to alter this state of affairs, nurses must stop being token instruments of physicians, and actively develop a separate, self-directing philosophy that is in accord with the goals and purposes of feminism.

While Ashley's view is perhaps more extreme than most, she is by no means alone in her accusation of female suppression. Lovell specifically accuses, the male-dominated medical profession of conspiring to "use and abuse" women in their roles as wives and as nurses. She states, "If the physician, in his role as dominant of the dominants, is a 'man among men,' then the nurse is 'the perfect woman'." Her central thesis is that women have historically been dominated and controlled in order to further the careers, finances, and personal goals of medical men. Like Ashley, she urges nurses to break loose from this imposed restraint.

Greenleaf considers the economic effects of belonging to a female occupation. She presents clear data regarding the degree to which nurses suffer economically by failing to receive "equal pay for equal worth." For example, in the 1977, Department of Labor rating of job complexity, a factor used in salary determinations, the job of staff nurse in a medical setting was rated as less complex than those of a physician's assistant or laboratory technician in a veterinary service. Greenleaf also believes this undervaluing of nurses' work is directly attributable to an androcentric ideology that defines men's domain as the public sphere and man's work as essential and difficult; women's sphere is the home, and women's work is unimportant to the greater society.

**Coordination in Critical Care**

The previous section has briefly reviewed some of the social norms and organizational characteristics that influence the role of the critical care nurse. Although the work group in most settings may be very cohesive, supportive, and efficient, it does not actually constitute a team in the strict sense. Characteristics of the specific unit and specific hospital may be significant determinants of how well the nurses and physicians work together.

In addition, explanations for the fact that the roles of coordinator and advocate are not formally assigned to, nor assumed by, nurses were discussed. These included a persistence of the historical image of nurses as handmaidens to physicians, prejudice and economic repression secondary to sex stereotyping, and lack of recognition as a profession, which is attributed to functional redundancy. Although important and relevant, these situational forces are not sufficient to counteract the persistent notions of nurses as coordinators and advocates. In fact, those experienced in critical care may well question why, given these factors, many nurses in many units *do* act as coordinators at times and are *able* to advocate effectively for some patients.

The answer to our dilemma may lie in a closer look at some of the other aspects of the critical care nurse's day-to-day responsibilities. For the purposes of our discussion, let us consider the care of a patient in an ICU in a large urban hospital. At the very least, the patient will have

primary physicians, dieticians, laboratory technicians, and one or two allied professionals, such as a respiratory therapist and social worker, involved in his care. All of these individuals need to obtain information about the patient, have access to the patient, and transmit information back to the other caregivers. The gatekeeper or controller of these interactions has to be the nurse. The nurse at the bedside is the logical individual to answer questions about the patient, help plan a trip to x-ray, schedule a breathing treatment, and receive information intended for one of the other caregivers. Aside from simply being there to discuss plans with others, the nurse has the broadest data base from which to operate. It is the nurse who is there to observe the effects of the medication ordered by the physician, evaluate what time of day is best for a breathing treatment, know what preparations are necessary prior to a CAT scan, and know how the patient tolerated a new diet. If the patient has consultants involved in his care, it is the nurse who must integrate the consultants' orders and recommendations with the orders of the primary physician. Because the nurse is responsible for the "whole" patient, he or she is the person most likely to identify a need or problem that is not being addressed by anyone.

Coordination of these activities, plans, and communications is not really an optional activity. In fact, it is something that must be done if one is to get through the day! It is only a small transition from coordinating the activities of eight hours to coordinating the course of the patient's entire ICU stay. Experienced nurses quite naturally make this transition, resulting in an easier job for everyone else and better care for the patient. It is problematic only when the coordination has to be done very overtly and others must alter their plans in a significant fashion. Under such circumstances, the nurse's formal status and the lack of official recognition of the coordinator role are likely to produce conflict.

A similar analysis applies to the advocate role. The presence of nurses 24 hours a day and patients' willingness to talk with them about their concerns, hopes, and fears have previously been mentioned as factors supporting nurses' suitability for the advocacy role. Since the critical care nurse is literally at the bedside on a continuous basis, he or she cannot help but observe and participate in all of the patient's physiological and emotional reactions. It is the nurse who is available to help the patient who has been told that he must return to surgery, have an amputation, or give up his job because of his heart condition. It is the nurse with whom the patient talks when he refuses a treatment. It is the nurse who is at the bedside when the family arrives and asks, "How is he." It is the nurse who implements orders and evaluates care when the patient cannot speak for himself and has no family.

The above-mentioned situations make it clear that one must be an advocate in order to provide nursing care. Unlike the surgeon, who operates for a specific pathology, the cardiologist, whose purpose is to prescribe medical treatment for heart disease, the internist, who cures or treats a specific disorder and its sequelae, *caring for the person* is the nurse's reason for existence. There is no way to do this without entering into the patient's world and assuming the patient's wishes, hopes, and fears. It is extremely difficult to respond to the patient who refuses surgery, states the medicine isn't helping, or says he doesn't want to live if he can't work, without being committed to working towards the patient's own goals.

Families expect nurses to intervene on behalf of patients. Perhaps one of the most difficult situations for the nurse-advocate to deal with is when the family approaches the nurse with questions and doubts about the appropriateness of continuing treatment or outright requests for the termination of life-support therapies. While the nurse may try to redirect the family's questions and concerns to the physician, the obligation to address expressed needs and wishes remains. The terrible, self-imposed burden of omniscience carried by the physician leaves him with the conviction that he already knows what is in the patient's best interest. Other caregivers, such as respiratory therapists or social workers, may be able to neatly identify such concerns as being outside of their purview. Nurses have no such avenues to relieve them from dealing with patient and family concerns; nor can they simply escape by leaving the situation.

A specific example of this all-too-common situation may further clarify the dilemma of the nurse advocate. Consider the case of a 70year-old patient who has a history of chronic lung disease and metastatic prostate cancer. The patient is followed by a pulmonary specialist for his lung disease and an oncologist for his cancer. He came to the ICU when he developed a urinary tract infection which progressed to septic shock. He is intubated and on a respirator. An infectious disease specialist is the consultant advising on antibiotic regimens. The intensivist, or medical chief of the ICU, is directing his medical care in the unit.

The ICU nurse is likely to receive communication from the patient's wife and children that is based on their understanding of the prognosis and therapy of the illness, their understanding of what the physicians have said, and their questions, doubts, and satisfaction with the patient's care. In addition to communicating about matters related to the patient's illness and medical care, families also, over time, share information about other topics—for example, what the patient's life was like prior to the illness; the plans, goals, and hopes this illness has interrupted; identification of the decision makers in the family; past discussions regarding the patient's wishes for prolonged life support therapies; projections of what the patient would want.

Families do not often overtly ask the nurse to intervene in what they perceive as medical decisions. This probably reflects the public's view of the nurse as the physician's employee and helper. The nurse does, however, use the data communicated by the family to generate a diagnosis of patient/family problems and needs. Once these needs are identified, courses of action are indicated. In the same way that the nurse might determine that the patient is becoming dehydrated and take measures to correct this problem, the nurse must find a way to address patient or family distress—regardless of whether the family has overtly asked for nursing intervention.

There are many options potentially available to the nurse—for example, simply sharing the family's communication with others; getting answers from the physician to transmit back to the family; arranging meetings between physician and family; helping the family to ask their questions or raise their concerns with physicians or other caregivers; instituting a plan to enable consistency in the manner in which others interact with the family. Doing nothing is rarely acceptable. Repeated contact with the family, repeated questions and expressions of distress, and the reality of having to participate in care that is inadequate, unsatisfactory, or simply not wanted generate feelings which, in turn, provide the nurse with powerful motivations for advocacy attempts.

In order to fulfill the role of the nurse, a means of dealing with the perceived needs and wishes of patients and families must be found. As with the role of coordinator, the extent to which the nurse attempts to enact this role in a formal, overt manner, the skill with which it is performed, and the relationships established with other caregivers often determine whether the nurse will be successful or generate resentment in others and fail to accomplish the purpose.

## CONCLUSION

Hospitals in the 1990s face an on-going crisis brought about by economic, political, and social conditions in the larger society. First medical care establishment has been illness-oriented, and both the insurance industry and health care programs have supported this priority. Some shifts toward prevention, health maintenance programs, and ambulatory care have occurred, but these efforts remain in the minority. Hospital care is expensive, and because of funding cuts, increasing numbers of patients, especially the poor, have no access to medical care.

Second, the population characteristics of hospital patients are changing. Patients are older, with more complex health problems, and are sicker at every age when they arrive at a hospital for care. Prospective payment or managed care systems imposed by insurers, including Medicare, reduce the length of hospital stays. Consequently, patients are discharged earlier with more illness needs and less independence than ever before. The spread of acquired immune deficiency syndrome (AIDS) and other communicable diseases like hepatitis and drug-resistant tuberculosis have revolutionized the interpersonal and physical health care environments in all settings.

Third, hospitals in all areas are increasingly called on to provide comprehensive services, including those requiring highly specialized and technical equipment that may become obsolete very rapidly. These trends are expensive and require large numbers of highly competent personnel, particularly nurses.

Fourth, a nursing shortage of unprecedented proportions is being felt throughout the world. The shortage is a result of an increased demand for nurses, a diminishing supply, and an attrition of working nurses from the profession. Many reasons have been proposed for this shortage: declining numbers of college-aged young people; expanding career opportunities for women; fewer women attracted to nursing; increasing numbers of nurses leaving the field for other careers; nursing's being perceived as low in status, income potential, and employment benefits; the realities of unattractive work schedules; and the risks of hospital environments. On the other hand, current economic conditions and rising unemployment of both men and women in many other occupations have made nursing increasingly attractive. Applications to nursing schools have increased in the past few years, and enrollments are up. Characteristics of graduate nurses and their career paths in the future may be more and more diverse and interesting.

Finally, hospitals have lost nurses to newer settings. Nurses who traditionally worked in hospitals have been attracted to the benefits of home health care and out-patient clinics. Changes in Medicare reimbursement to hospitals, introduced in 1983, have encouraged physicians to discharge patients earlier from hospitals. Much of traditional illness care has shifted from hospitals to home and clinic settings. Nurses have left hospitals to work in these environments.

Linda Aiken disputes the premise that the nursing shortage reflects declining numbers. She points out that although actual enrollments in nursing schools have declined some 25 percent since 1984, the numbers of graduates exceeds the numbers of nurses retiring, thus reflecting an increase in the size of the actual pool of nurses. Further, 80 percent of nurses are employed in nursing, a high percentage for a predominantly female occupation. The high turnover in hospital nursing positions, Aiken believes, reflects widespread dissatisfaction among nurses with hospital employment. However, since most nurses who resign hospital positions take a job in another hospital, nurse resignations and hospital vacancy rates do not reflect an actual nursing shortage.

Any discussion of nursing practice in critical care requires an introduction to the setting, to the needs of the patient, and to the role of the nurse The practicing nurse in critical care settings is a participant in the most intimate life and death events that persons can experience in dealing with illness. Other medical groups share this domain with nursing. Physicians, clergy, physical and respiratory therapists, social workers, and hospital administrators are among the many professionals who interact with critically ill patients and their families in the modern hospital. But the characteristics of nursing practice in hospitals make the role of the nurse unique among the various professional groups that serve patients and their families. The particular skills, the persistence of caring, and the continuous round-the-clock presence of nurses in hospitals form a triad that renders nursing distinctive from other health groups.

Nurses may assume a special role with very ill patients in which direct and continuous support of physiological, emotional, social, and spiritual functions is provided.

Nurses may use a wide variety of skills and techniques to take care of patients. A problem-solving or nursing process approach is generally accepted by professional and educational groups; practice, licensing, and accrediting bodies; and the institutions where nursing is practiced as an appropriate framework for nursing practice and activities. This approach includes assessing and diagnosing patient problems, planning and goal setting for individual patient needs, intervening for each problem, and evaluating results. Pain and anxiety are examples of patient problems for which nurses might intervene. In hospitals, nurses might be involved in direct care of patients, management, teaching, research, or consultation regarding patient care. Nursing roles in hospitals may also encompass coordinating the multiple services involved in patient care.

The direct care nursing role in critical care settings involves assessing the complex interplay of illness or dysfunction of the individual as a physiologic and psychologic whole. The nurse may be considered an extension of the functions of a person unable to care for him- or herself. The patient crisis may be elective surgery, overwhelming infection, trauma, angina, or multiple system failure and coma. The nurse provides physical care and monitors vital functions including heart rate; blood pressure; skin integrity; bowel and bladder functions; nutritional, fluid, electrolyte, and mobility status; and mentation. The nurse assesses for abnormalities and takes action to help the patient return to normal function. For example, a nurse may increase intravenous fluids if a postoperative patient seems volume depleted, as evidenced by low urine output, rapid heart rate, low blood pressure, and poor skin turgor. On the other hand, a nurse may discontinue oral fluids or food in this same patient in the presence of abdominal distension and decreased bowel sounds. Critical care nurses, using parameters and "judgments" related to interacting factors, routinely titrate drip rates of very potent drugs that affect the heart, blood pressure, cardiac output, and blood sugar level. The special skills and experiences that the nurse possesses regarding normal responses to the intrusion of illness provide a basis for judgment. Nursing judgment is difficult to define or quantify, but remains a core competency for any effective nurse in an acute care setting, especially a critical care nurse.

The direct care role makes the nurse a "patient extender." If the patient is paralyzed, the nurse turns the patient to prevent pneumonia and puts all limbs through a passive range of motion to prevent contracture and muscle wasting. If the patient is blind, the nurse will describe the environment of the room so the patient can walk safely. The nursing role goes beyond direct care and involves managing individual responses to illness, rehabilitation, or dying. The nurse may assist the patient and family to assess self-care motivation and potential, to acquire or develop special skills or adaptive equipment, and to obtain reimbursement for acute and long-term care.

In the intensive care unit the nurse collects and monitors vast amounts of detailed data. This monitoring is continuous and occurs in rapidly changing situations. These judgments require anticipation of subtle changes and decision making, interpretations, intervention, and evaluation in complex situations. The outcomes of these decisions may have life and death potential for patients. The decision making may occur in units that are inadequately staffed, organized, and managed and have little or no competent medical back-up. Further, the invasive and life-extending procedures that patients may experience may be perceived as dehumanizing by the nurse and others. When realistic expectation of recovery is lost and the patient's deterioration prolonged, nurses may experience extreme stress at the loss of hope. One nurse expressed the pain of "taking care of dead people. I just can't do it anymore."

The illnesses that place patients in critical care settings are crisis events, often sudden, painful, and excruciating in their impact on patient and family. For example, the crisis of head injury after an automobile accident may be complicated by pregnancy, old age, chronic illness, or AIDS.

Decision making by the patient and family is required during a period of high stress, limited knowledge, and consequent dependence on the judgment of medical and nursing personnel. The diagnostic and treatment regimes offered to patients are often ambiguous, and the outcomes may be painful, expensive, and disfiguring. Patients often experience a cycle of incremental decision making, ambiguity, and ambivalence. They encounter machines, procedures, and technology that seem like experimentation or science fiction. They may sense a climate of chaotic unreality, over which they feel no control. The endurance and the outcomes of such experiences are highly stressful for patients and family members. No wonder patients are highly susceptible to stress-related illness such as stress ulcers and psychoses in critical care settings.

The critical care setting has also been shown to be very stressful for hospital staff, and the rate of burnout for physicians and nurses is very high in these areas. Joan L. Stehle, Menzies, and Holsclaw have noted that nursing in general is seen as stressful because of patient suffering and death, heavy demands, frightening tasks, and disturbing relationships with patients. Nurses feel impotent, especially when they are unable to restore patients to well-being. Although critical care settings have been persistently identified as stressful, Friedman and Strauss have noted that factors identified as stressors for some ICU nurses are identified as sources of satisfaction, challenge, and increased staff intimacy and morale by others. Koumans and Strauss have identified the following particular stressors for nurses in critical care settings: rapid turnover of staff, intensity of emotions in interpersonal situations, complicated machinery, narrow patient care focus, great responsibility, conflict with administration, and crisis atmosphere. The great variability among these factors indicates the complexity of the critical care setting for nurses, patients, and others. Interestingly, these observations were made in the 1960s, before the rapid increase in technology and specialization.

Altruism and caretaking have been persistent themes throughout the history of nursing. The roots of nursing altruism have been traced to nineteenthcentury reform movements, religion, and traditional women's roles. Susan Reverby has explored the "central dilemma of nursing: the order to care in a society that refuses to value caring" her thesis maintains that the order to care was rooted in the duty ascribed to feminine roles. This duty carried obligations but not rights. Nursing therefore must forge a link between altruism and autonomy in order to have "caring-with-autonomy" and "a way of life that includes serving others without being subservient". Nursing professionalism, the economics of nursing as a predominantly female occupation, the history of both the proposed and actual educational requirements for entry into nursing practice, and the work settings where nursing is practiced are a few of the issues that are influenced by the altruistic roots of nursing. Little attention has been given by scholars to the influence of these issues on the motivation, self-concept, and career choices of nurses and the ways in which various nurses relate to medicine, the hospital, and the larger society.

Contemporary critical care settings engender great potential for loss of human integrity, self-worth, and self-control for patients, family members, and nurses. There is also great potential for meaningful human interaction and intimacy. The nurse is in a position to assist the patient and family to humanize that environment and crisis situation, and perhaps gain some control over life, illness, or death in the hostile hospital environment and create the sort of climate that families and friends might forge in a home setting for an ill loved one.

The central features of the contemporary critical care setting include constant nursing care of complicated patients in highly technical, increasingly specialized, rapidly changing, and complex environments. The moral, social, and ethical dimensions of decision making in these environments are not clear, and the nurse is bound through interpersonal and professional role functions in a pivotal relationship with patient, family, physician, and hospital. Scholars are only beginning to explore the characteristics and dimensions of the stresses and perhaps the satisfactions of these relationships. How distinctive critical care nursing is as a specialty and how representative it is of the discipline as a whole remain questions to be tested relative to traditional roles and to changes affecting nursing and contemporary practice.

Nursing as a discipline and nurses as individuals remain obscure in written histories. Hilberman documents a chronological history of critical care units with only a passing mention of nurses. Starr traces the history of the health industry with only an incidental reference to nursing, the largest group of health care workers in the country. Dorothy Marlow's pediatric nursing textbook gives a history of child care with a list of dates and events of importance, without listing any nursing event or primary sources. Interestingly, by the sixth edition in 1988, the role of the nurse is discussed throughout the section. Nursing is presumed to exist in the shadow of political events and medical accomplishments.

Traditional nursing and medical histories demonstrate class, racial, and sexist biases and problems with primary source materials in addition to their regional biases and their neglect of nursing as an occupation of significance. The documented histories are chronologies of the activities of middle- and upper-class women, most often told from the perspective of institutional or medical priorities. The primary source materials available pertaining to nursing – for example, the written documentation of nursing school curricula, records of professional nursing organizations, and records of medical treatment – do not reflect the essence of nursing practice. The life experiences and personal commitments of individual nurses remain as obscure as the dimensions of their interactions with patients. Even medical and nursing histories that use primary source materials and portray the unique experience of individuals and minorities are often biased to region.

The history of nursing specialty organizations have also remained obscure. In 1988, however, the Association of Critical Care Nurses awarded a grant to conduct research for the purpose of writing a history of the organization.

As G. Grob notes, social history approaches to the history of disease and medicine can reveal fundamental values in our society "and reflect the size and structure of the population, the social structure, technology, and living and cultural pattern in society". In recent years social historians and others have reduced many of the kinds of biases that have been discussed above. Further, they have begun to ask more appropriate questions and to acknowledge the limitations of existing data. This trend has been furthered by interests in the nurse as worker, as female, as hospital employee, and as participant in grassroots health care. Still, the practicing nurse is less visible in written histories than the bureaucratic education and practice organizations.

As an occupational history of a largely female group, the story of the evolution of nursing, particularly critical care nursing, provides a view of changing women's roles since World War II. It also provides a perspective on the ways in which nurses and nursing have interacted with individuals, other occupations, and institutions – notably, patients, medicine, and hospitals respectively. Nursing has been the persistent human factor in the evolution of critical care units in hospitals. Nurses are the largest group of workers in hospitals and are the only hospital employees with consistent, round-the-clock contact with patients. Hence, the history of critical care nursing reflects the many changes in hospital care of patients that have occurred since World War II. Most visible among these changes have been the emergence of medical specialization and the increased use of highly technical equipment for diagnosis, treatment, and direct patient care at the bedside.

A study of the characteristics of nursing practice in ICU settings reveals information about the ways in which nurses, patients, and others respond to the complex, stressful, and highly technical critical care environment. A study of critical care nursing is also a valuable source of information about the interactions between nurses and patients and their families, physicians, and others; the actual nursing care delivered; and the ethical dimensions of critical care practice.

The structure and organization of contemporary critical care units are predictable and reflect external standards and regulations. The nursing literature reflects a young, self-absorbed discipline largely concerned with professional standards, education, leadership, and performance issues. The human, interpersonal experience of nursing practice and the knowledge inherent in practice have received less attention.

Dolores Garlo studied the legal dimensions of the evolution of critical care nursing, and proposed that the application of technology resulted in the critical care nursing specialty. The distinctiveness of critical care nursing and its representation of nursing as a general discipline await description. Certainly the nurse, the patient, and a high concentration of technology and equipment define the critical care setting. R. Vreeland and G. L. Ellis have made a significant observation about the paradoxical nature of the ICU nurse's situation, where warmth and sympathy are expected together with objectivity and assertiveness.

Our motivation for studying the history of critical care nursing practice is rooted in merging realities. It seems that nurses do everything and are constantly taking on more. The challenges to accomplish "everything" are hypnotic, and the costs are insidious. Stress effects, mechanistic performance or even incompetence, and "burnout" are a few of the very real outcomes. Also very real and powerful are the intimacies between nurses and patients and/or their families in these highly stressful settings. An energy potential, almost like a stretched rubber band, can permeate these interactions.

We know that nurses make a difference to patients and families and to their own humanity when they intervene in the debilitating, dehumanizing, and ethically demanding situations that can occur as a consequence of "high-tech" treatment. We have seen nurses take control of the details of these settings and empower hopelessly ill or dying patients and their families to make choices and get some control and humanity back into their lives. Other persons, especially physicians and chaplains, are involved, but nurses are with patients constantly. We know that these interactions with patients are intimate and powerful and at the core of the skills, attitudes, and values that define nursing practice: competence, caring, and commitment. That story of nursing is not reported in any of the literature of nursing or other disciplines.

Our interest in social history, especially women's history, since nursing has been so predominantly female, precipitated the second reality. The traditional histories, We looked at did not reflect the human experience of care taking, both because of the narrow selection of sources and because of the priorities of the writers.

R. H. Abzug describes the impact of oral interviews with American liberators of the concentration camps: "they afford us a window on the way men and women act and think when faced with the unimaginable suffering of others. The deep compassion and sometimes the limits of vision displayed...pointed to important ambivalences about facing the Holocaust and its victims...and the immediate and long-range impact of their discoveries on the public mind.

The purpose of this book is to explore the evolution and contemporary practice of critical care nursing from the perspective of the practicing nurse through history. The following questions will be explored:

- What has been the experience of nurses in critical care units during a period of increasing specialization and the use of rapidly changing and complex technology.
- What is the essence of nursing practice in critical care settings.
- What are the practice issues and the range of nurses' responses to the ethical dimensions of critical care nursing practice.

This chapter has described critical care nurses as young, female, and educated in college or university settings. They are attracted to what may be an especially stressful setting by the challenges and opportunities for learning and developing their competencies. They share other nurses' susceptibilities to the negative effects of inadequate staffing, lack of pay for comparable worth, conflicts of loyalty between patient care and institutional goals, and lack of respect from physicians.

Like all nurses, the critical care nurse is oriented towards caring for the whole person and the wellness state. The uniqueness of the nursing role is derived from the unique combination of skills and abilities utilized in caring for patients 24 hours a day, rather than the specific tasks performed. All nurses are potentially capable of developing special relationships with their patients; in the ICU, this potential is enhanced by the patient's total dependence upon the nurse's caring and competence.

On the one hand, this special relationship contributes to the critical care nurse's attempts to act as advocate and coordinator. At the same time, the norms and values of the ICU environment prevent the nurse from gaining the formal rights necessary to fulfill these roles. The nurse can deal with this dilemma in several ways.

The nurse may attempt to deal with problems in an open and mature fashion, focusing on the patient's needs and confronting conflicts as they occur. This is clearly the most desirable approach, although it often precipitates additional stress. The nurse who perceives him/herself to be a competent professional, with appropriate goals based on identified patient needs and wishes, will not tolerate behavior on the part of others that denigrates the nurse's status or appears contrary to the patient's best interest. If the nurse disagrees with, or is concerned about, the care provided by others, he or she will intervene. Such an approach will obviously generate reactions from others, which will be based on their perceptions of the appropriateness of the nurse's intervention, the nurse's "proper" role in the unit, and the nurse's specific behaviors. This may result in everyone's gaining a better understanding of mutual goals, priorities, or points of difference, which may eventually produce a healthier working relationship. Or, it may result in heightened conflict and reinforced misperceptions. The fact that ICUs are staffed by young caregivers, who are not only struggling to establish their professional identities but are often not secure in their personal identities, makes this an all too frequent outcome.

The "doctor-nurse game" is another option for a nurse who is trying to achieve his/her goal. Stein coined this term to describe a mode of communication to which doctors and nurses are socialized. In this variation on sex-based stereotypes, the nurse assumes a naive, unsophisticated demeanor in approaching the physician, the wise healer, who will assist in her plight—that is, will do what she wants for her patient. The object of the game is to have the nurse make a recommendation to the physician without appearing to do so. The physician is thus able to utilize the nurse as an expert consultant without actually asking advice, which would seriously threaten his image of omnipotence. This type of behavior is often the path of least resistance; it provides a quick way for the nurse to obtain the orders she needs for the patient, get a new IV started, or get the house officer to talk with the patient's family. However, it also demeans both parties, and reinforces a distorted image of the nurse as a helpless female and the physician as an omniscient being.

When facing a conflict, another appropriate option is to refer the problem to a higher authority. As members of the hospital's formal bureaucratic heirarchy, nurses are more likely to exercise this option than physicians, who may be more reluctant to appeal to others for help. The importance of having a supportive supervisor, and the deleterious effects of not having this resource available, are attested to by the stress studies mentioned earlier. Both Bailey and Huckaby found unresponsive nursing leadership and communication problems with supervisors to be among the most significant sources of stress. Inability or reluctance to appeal to higher authority is an unfortunate situation in that it eliminates an effective means of dealing with conflict. Referring disagreements to a higher level removes the issue from the bedside and assists in focusing on the issues themselves, rather than the personalities involved. Relocating the conflict frees staff nurses and physicians from interpersonal tensions that can hamper effective functioning, and is a valuable way to prevent disagreements from affecting patient care.

Another way for nurses to maximize their ability to control the situation is by utilizing their unlimited informal power. After a few years of experience in an ICU, the nurse becomes a system expert. He or she learns how to get "stat" lab results, which medications are stocked, the preferences and routines of senior attending physicians, and how the equipment works. In addition, the experienced nurse is quite knowledgeable about the usual effects of particular therapies, the usual course of a disease, recommended medication dosages, and other aspects of patient care that the young house officer has simply not yet had a chance to learn. Having this knowledge is a source of tremendous power for the nurse, enabling her to choose between help ing the inexperienced physician or letting him flounder and learn the hard way. The nurse's choice is often influenced by the quality of previous interactions, the individual physician involved, professional security, and the other's willingness to request and receive help from a nurse.

The descriptions of these interactional styles are not meant to type-cast critical care nurses; they are meant to demonstrate how the issues discussed earlier in this chapter affect the relationships between the nurse and other caregivers. If there is a lesson to be learned from this analysis of critical care nursing, it is that the problems are more complex than they initially appear. The critical care nurse is a product of the history of nursing, the struggles of women in our society, the modern intensive care unit environment, and, most importantly, the conflicts and positive relationships with other care providers.

# Chapter 2

# History of Critical Care Nursing

## INTRODUCTION

Critical care nursing is a post- World War II phenomenon. Its development paralleled the rise of medical specialization and the rapid emergence of complex medical technology. According to N. M. Simon, the modern intensive care unit (ICU) concept owes its development to three major forces. First, the recovery room experience in the 1940s and 1950s has shown to medicine and nursing the advantage of intensive and continual surveillance, by nurses, of very ill patients. Second, the progressive patient care concept proposed by hospital planners determined that patients in hospitals would be grouped according to the amount and intensity of nursing care required, in facilities designed to meet their special needs. Third, an evolving complex technology that permitted more ambitious surgical procedures required increasingly complex postoperative surveillance and nursing care.

The direct antecedent of the intensive care unit was the postoperative recovery room, which came into common use in the 1950s. Prerequisite and concurrent developments included those as diverse as antiseptic surgery, X-ray, blood transfusion, the hypodermic needle and syringe, the ventilator, cardiopulmonary resuscitation, various types of anesthesia, and drugs for pain relief, immunization, and antibiotics. Treatment of battle casualties during World War II and the Korean and Vietnam wars produced new surgical techniques and treatment and supported the growth of critical care nursing as a specialty. Factors as varied as the role of women in the military and the emergence of the helicopter for triage and evacuation of the wounded for treatment elsewhere further refined the role of the critical care nurse

The post-World War II trend toward hospital staff employment for nurses coincided with the boom in hospital building precipitated by funds for hospital construction . Specialization continued within medicine, paralleling new technologies and developments in cardiac surgery and arteriography, such as the heart-lung machine. Chemotherapeutic drugs and radiation in the treatment of cancer also developed during this period. The emergence of Medicare and Medicaid in the 1960s coincided with the struggle for equal rights for women and minority groups, and influenced health care availability and access for these groups. The development of oral contraceptives ushered in an era of changed sexual mores and family patterns. These events coincided with concerns about nuclear destruction, the pollution of the environment, and electronic developments such as the transistor and the twentieth-century microchip. The recent emergence of acquired immune deficiency syndrome (AIDS) has presented the threat of a major global epidemic that as yet has no effective treatment or cure. The health care industry, reflecting society, has only begun to confront the enormous implications of this disease.

Developments in nursing education and practice may be examined in the context of the aforementioned rapid social and technological changes, which have had impacts on health and illness. After World War II, money was increasingly available for nursing education, and nurses were assured employment in increasing numbers of hospitals and various health agencies. In the 1970s, 1980s, and 1990s, hospitals became more specialized and costly, but simultaneously there was a trend toward health promotion, improved nutrition and exercise, and outpatient care.

Critical care nursing developed during the phase of medical specialization in the 1960s. By 1970, hospitals were the third largest industry in the United States, surpassed only by the steel and automobile industries. The coronary care unit, established in 1962, greatly improved patients' chances of surviving heart attacks, and nurses with specialized knowledge were required to care for these patients. Just as nurses practiced in recovery rooms and specialized surgical intensive care units, the coronary care unit nurses "nursed" in another new setting with refined skills and broadened scopes of practice that perhaps often challenged existing nurse practice acts. As new specialties, including neurosurgery, organ transplantation, burn treatment, and trauma care, developed, specialized intensive care units emerged to care for patients in these units. Nursing was designed to support the physical and psychosocial needs of patients moving through periods of crisis resolution toward recovery, rehabilitation, or death.

The common thread through this trend toward specialization was the practice of expert nursing for twenty-four hours a day, in increasingly complex environments. A specialty organization, the Association of Critical Care Nurses, emerged in the 1970s. This group published a professional journal, defined critical care practice and education standards, conducted national meetings, provided regional and local workshops and chapter organizations, promoted a certification examination for critical care nurses, and sponsored critical care nursing research.

Critical care nursing cannot be understood in isolation from nursing as a professional discipline. While geographical and specialization designations such as the emergency room, the coronary care unit, or the intensive care unit may imply critical care, the distinctiveness of critical care nursing awaits description. In fact, little scholarship exists to indicate whether critical care nursing represents a concentration of nursing practice as a whole or reflects something innovative and different Further, the impact of specialization and the rapid influx of technological change on nursing practice has gained the attention of few researchers. The uniqueness of nursing practice in these settings has received even less attention.

Similarly, as in nursing in general, little is known about the human dimensions of the practice of a critical care nurse. The critical care nurse lives twenty-four hours a day, seven days a week, in highly stressful, intellectually demanding, and rapidly changing environments, with and for patients with multiple needs. This patient population is sicker and older than before, with more complex health problems requiring a variety of interventions. Further, critical care nurses are now at risk of exposure to life-threatening diseases like AIDS, hepatitis, and tuberculosis and injury from toxic products and processes such as x-rays in the environment. The involvement of the nurse with the patient, the patient's family and friends, the physicians, and other health care personnel may exemplify a model of communication and practice that is unique. Little is known about the motivation of critical care nurses for involving themselves in these situations and assuming these risks.

There is, unfortunately, little scholarship on this aspect of nursing practice. Certainly the conflict in values and beliefs and the ethical and moral dimensions of nursing practice in these settings merit further study. Finally, a scholarly caution is in order. The statements above can describe nurse-patient interactions not traditionally described as critical care, by nurses not defined as critical care nurses. The designation of critical care nursing as distinctive and unique, or as representative of the discipline as a whole, remains a question for study. The examination of the development of critical care nursing practice that follows may help illuminate these questions.

## History of Critical Care Nursing

A formal comprehensive history of critical care nursing has not been written. Most discussions of the development of either critical care nursing or the critical care unit have addressed dimensions of three closely associated phenomena: the rapid emergence of a highly technical medical environment, medical and nursing specialization, and the associated changes in hospital organization and personnel. These developments have been relatively recent and change has occurred very rapidly.

The roots of medical technology and specialization have been traced to antiquity. Aristotle distinguished the arteries from the veins, and Galen noted that the arteries, when cut, always "gushed blood." He applied a tie, or tourniquet, to arteries to stop bleeding . If we accept technology as "applied science, a technical method for achieving a practical purpose", the use of the tourniquet may represent the application of a new technology in ancient Greece. As J. D. Bolter points out, tools epitomize the stages of human development; clay pottery, the clock, and the steam engine represent progressive stages of development. To this sequence Bolter adds the computer, predicting that future intellectual efforts will involve the use of computers.

In analyzing technology as a shaping force in contemporary society, I. L. Bennett, Jr. notes that technology is often defined as the practical application of scientific research. Although this assessment is limited, it is true that public concern with problems created by technological change such as the deterioration of family life, alienation, boredom, anxiety, drug use, and mental illness often focuses blame on the scientific community. Further, the scientist may be seen as a culprit by people who fear the nuclear annihilation, pollution, extinction of plant and animal species, and dehumanization that are often associated with technological development.

New technologies may be classified as substitute or add-on technologies. New technology may substitute a better, more efficient way of accomplishing something previously possible or may add on or make possible something previously unknown. Most new medical technologies are add-ons. They accomplish something, at increased cost, that was not previously possible. However, they do not necessarily increase productivity in the health establishment or reduce cost to the consumer or to society. Furthermore, decisions about new medical technologies may be based on the technologies' perceived impact on lessening disability and pain and prolonging life or on access to decision makers about funding priorities.

According to Bennett, the medical establishment appears to deviate from adherence to the principle that market demand stimulates technological advances. Several factors seem to be at work in contributing to the reality that Lewis Thomas has described – that "in medicine, it is characteristic of technology that we do not count the cost, ever, even when the bills begin coming in". First, the consumer of medical technology is now the physician rather than the patient. It is the physician who orders hospitalization, diagnostic tests, surgery, and drugs. Second, the physician follows the concept of technological imperative – the belief that all physicians, patients, and hospitals should have available all the technologies of medicine, regardless of cost, priorities, or allocation of resources. The supplier creates the demand. Third, the reimbursement system for payment of medical costs historically has been less influenced by market forces than have other parts of the economy. Recent changes in Medicare reimbursement, however, suggest alterations from a system where the physician or hospital creates the demand, sets the cost, and guarantees payment .

Many thoughtful individuals in various disciplines have reflected on the meaning of the machine for quality of life issues that influence the interplay of individuals and the larger society and the planet. In his examination of the interplay of technical developments in Western civilization with aspects of the social, scientific, and political milieu, Lewis Mumford describes the clock as the key machine of the modern age. Once the technical development of the clock was given substance in the ordered monastic tradition "time-keeping passed into time-serving and time-accounting and timerationing. Time replaced eternity as the measure of human action".

Alvin Toffler and John Naisbitt have provided commentaries on the evolutionary and revolutionary changes predicted in the transition from an industrial to an information world. Because of their articulation of issues and their media visibility, both men have had an impact on the larger society and on scholarly and applied work in this area. Toffler describes a third new era of human existence, a synthesizing, future oriented era replacing the agricultural and industrial eras that preceded it. The trend is toward global, open, multi-option, emerging realities. Naisbitt similarly describes an emerging society that is being restructured in profoundly technical ways. The economy is now based more on information than on industrialization. New technology imposes a human response at each phase. Economic considerations are focused more on global and long-term considerations than on national and short-term issues. Centralization, institutional help, representative democracy, and formal hierarchies are being replaced by decentralization, self-help, participatory democracy, and networking.

According to Fritzof Capra, society faces a transitional crisis similar to the change in concepts and ideas from the mechanistic views of Descartes and Newton to the more holistic and ecological view that occurred in physics as a result of the exploration of the atomic and sub-atomic world in the early twentieth century. Capra proposes a new paradigm, or vision of reality, that would include the "emerging systems view of life, mind, consciousness, and evolution; the corresponding holistic approach to health and healing. The integration of western and eastern approaches to psychology and psychotherapy; a new conceptual framework for economics and technology; and an ecological and feminist perspective which is spiritual in its ultimate nature and will lead to profound changes in our societal and political structure".

J. P. Martino proposes a decision-making model of technological forecasting in which methodological and statistical techniques are incorporated into a decision-making framework for use by engineers, scientists, and administrators. The significance of this model, in the context of this discussion, is the fact that such a framework is intended to command the realities of present and future technologies.

According to Alfred North Whitehead, the relationship between the time span of major cultural change and the life span of individuals determines the nature of education. As long as the time span of cultural change exceeds the life span of individuals, education can be considered the transmission of knowledge. In essence, what individuals learn in their youth remains valid for the rest of their lives. In the twentieth century time span of cultural change is considerably shorter than the human life span. Thus, training and education must prepare individuals to face a variety of conditions. Whitehead's observations have direct application in the area of enlarging medical and nursing technologies.

As A. W. Mathies Jr. has described, profound changes in medical education and practice have occurred as a result of emerging lifesupport technologies. Early attempts in the 1940s to assist premature infants with the new techniques of oxygen administration and the use of the antibiotic chloramphenical resulted in retrolental fibroplasia and gray baby syndrome respectively. These iatrogenic problems actively improved assessment techniques, research protocols, and methods of data collection. Varieties and amounts of data obtained increased dramatically. Large amounts of data also became available as space technology was directed to human health problems. Physicians came to be assisted by specialized engineers, technicians, respiratory therapists, and nurses who provided observations and data that required new models of assessment and analysis.

Mathies cites three structural outcomes of rapidly emerging technologies in medicine. First was the problem-oriented record as a systematic approach to medical management. Its components included the data base, the problem list, the initial plan, and the progress report. POMR facilitated the utilization of large amounts of information by the many individuals caring for a patient over time. Second, sub-specialities developed in critical care. As machines become more complex, engineers, computer scientists, and technicians with special competence in the care of machines were required in care settings. Physicians, nurses, and therapists were trained to interface these specialties in the management of critically ill patients. Critical care services required a multidisciplinary team approach to care. Third, life-support technology forced a rethinking of medical curricula. Content on humanism and ethics was included in medical education. Veatch concurs on factors that resulted from life-support technology. Students were exposed to content on death and dying, human behavior, family-patient relationships, medical ethics, and philosophy in education and practice areas of the medical school curricula.

The literature in critical care nursing in the decade of the 1980s reflected concerns about the particular outcomes of high technology on both nurses and patients in the critical care setting. Specialty and general nursing literature have reported frequently on strategies for coping, monitoring, or adopting new technologies such as dialysis, coronary care, computers, and new machines and monitors. As critical care units have become more common, the specific issues of touch, empathy, and stress, and human problems caused by the highly technical critical care environment, have become more apparent in the literature.

The stress effects of critical care settings have been increasingly recognized. Patients, their families, and nurses are influenced by many factors related to the environment and treatment options in critical care. Stress has been recognized as an outcome of highly invasive and technical treatment since the early 1950s. I. L. Janis study of the effects of stress on patients confronted with the unknown dangers of surgery found that careful, appropriate preoperative communication that allowed the patient to rehearse the danger situation mentally could greatly enhance postoperative adjustment. R. J. Vanson, B. M. Katz, and K. Krekeler reported significant stress effects in patients who witnessed invasive, technical procedures on other patients in a coronary care unit (CCU). Auditory and visual stimuli that increase stress effects in patients who witnessed the routine CCU procedure of Swan-Ganz catheter and pacemaker insertion and cardioversion may be reduced by providing glass-partitioned or private rooms.

V. S. Wilson study of stressors related to patients' psychologic responses to the surgical ICU found that over 50 percent of the subjects had an impaired psychologic response while in the ICU. One third of the sample experienced hallucinations, especially visual, without loss of orientation. Too much noise, losing track of time, hearing doctors or nurses talk about rather than to the patient, and being examined by several doctors and nurses were the most significant stressors that impaired healthy coping. Wilson recommends measures to prevent or minimize excessive stressors such as decreasing ICU environmental noise levels by reducing alarms and ventilator noise and providing private rooms; to detect and treat abnormal psychological responses through regular mental status examination of patients by nurses; and to assist the patient with excessive stress to re-adapt and maintain stability by explanations and continuous orientation by nurses.

Wilson and others have demonstrated strong correlations between sleep deprivation and impaired stress responses to the ICU environment. Sleep deprivation is difficult to test as an isolated variable because many factors impair stress responses, including the patient's age, severity of illness, psychological history, metabolic and drug factors, and the use of the cardiopulmonary bypass pump, as well as those environmental factors identified earlier by Wilson. Nonetheless, it is usually grouped with potential stressors and is considered a major factor in patient disorientation in ICU by most researchers.

Families, particularly spouses or significant others of patients in ICUs, experience a great deal of stress related to the crisis of hospitalization. As B. L. Fife notes, the serious illness or hospitalization of a family member presents a threatening crisis for a family unit. High levels of stress increase the family's vulnerability to the development of secondary problems related to economics, child behavior, child care, or disrupted role expectations. While some families have the resources to remain integrated during such a crisis, others experience temporary periods of disorganization, and still others are unable to remain intact.

The fear of losing a loved one through death and the stress of the strange and threatening environment of the CCU may precipitate a state of disequilibrium and crisis in family members. Stresses experienced by spouses of heart attack (acute myocardial infarction, AMI) patients in a coronary care unit were studied by M. S. Caplin and D. L. Sexton. The spouses and nurses ranked potential CCU stressors. While the two groups gave comparable responses with regard to highly ranked stressors, nurses over- or underestimated several stressors of importance to spouses. Spouses and nurses agreed on the high stress potential of fear of death, seeing the spouse sick, dealing with the ill spouse's reaction to the idea of having a heart attack, and not being informed about changes in the patient's condition.

Nurses underestimated the importance to the spouse of trying not to upset the ill person, thinking about difficulties when the patient gets home, not being able to sleep, being lonely, having difficulty concentrating, and the fact that parking was inconvenient and expensive. They overestimated the importance to spouses of indecision by doctors and nurses about diagnosis and lack of satisfaction with answers to questions by doctors and nurses. They also overestimated the importance to spouses of noisy alarms on the heart monitor, the care the patient was receiving, being asked to leave the room for a time, and hearing of another patient's death.

The major implication is for nurses to recognize and to address the stresses experienced by CCU patients and their spouses. Caplin and Sexton make the following recommendations. The nurse can help relieve some of the stresses of fear of spousal death by providing support and encouraging expression of feelings and fears. Continuity of care can help establish a relationship conducive to this kind of communication. Other family and clergy may assist in this process. The nurse should set aside time each day, away from the patient, to communicate with the spouse and to answer questions. Honest information presented in a simple and clear manner will help decrease anxiety. Visiting policies, especially, should be explained clearly at the time of admission. Spouses may be helped to sleep at night by being encouraged to call the CCU at bedtime to check on the partner. Finally, nurses can help by explaining clearly the normal adjustment to having a heart attack. Spouses may worry less if they recognize that the patient's disturbing behavior likely will be temporary.

Stress and coping in families of the critically ill are described by S. L. King and F. M. Gregor in their review of the literature. Although they acknowledge variability due to individual response, their evidence seems to indicate that stress increases when the person has no anticipatory preparation time, when exposure to stress is prolonged or multiple stressors occur concurrently, when events are ambiguous or uncertain, and when the exposure is to an event that involves a life event of importance, such as critical illness or survival. Families of critically ill patients experience high levels of stress not only because of the critical illness of the patient but because the illness or injury is usually unexpected, has an uncertain outcome, and has a critical phase that may be prolonged for days or weeks.

Sources of stress for family members are varied, but include fear of death, chronic pain, or permanent disability of the ill family member; uncertainty about the prognosis; loss of a strong family member; conflicts about the usual roles and obligations of work, dependence, and financial concerns; being away from home, staying in unfamiliar lodging, and loneliness; and the environment of unfamiliar caregivers, equipment, procedures, rules, smells, and sounds. If the patient is unconscious or on a ventilator, the family can experience additional sources of stress. The equipment is proof of the seriousness of the illness, and it prevents the patient from responding verbally. If the patient is unconscious, the uncertainty about outcome and fear of death are heightened.

Family members under stress report somatic symptoms, including the sleep disturbances of sleeping fewer hours and waking frequently, feeling depressed and unable to concentrate, restlessness, loss of appetite, and weight loss. These symptoms may reflect anxiety and/or ineffective coping, where coping is defined as "any efforts at stress management regardless of their effectiveness". Family members may utilize any number of mechanisms for managing stress. Some of the most common techniques are turning to others for support, remaining near the patient, information seeking, intellectualization, rehearsal, or review of the event, minimizing the situation, repetition, and hope.

The critical illness of a patient brings about multiple stressors for family members that they may manage in a variety of ways. Nurses may assist family members to utilize effective coping by helping them identify strategies that have been successful for them in the past and to capitalize on personal strengths and the resources available to them. Further, the nurse can reinforce or support their current effective coping efforts.

Many of the stresses of critical care nursing are related to the health care setting as a work environment. High levels of stress seem related to burnout in nurses, which is characterized by physical and emotional exhaustion and a loss of compassion and respect for clients. Burnout is a maladaptive reaction to occupational stressors and may also relate to turnover, absenteeism, serious on-the-job mistakes, and patient neglect. Burnout has been discussed in the nursing literature since 1978, and situational and social stressors that contribute to nurse burnout have been reported. These include occupational factors, the work setting, life event changes or personal stressors, and lack of social support. Questions remain about the impact of the intensity and frequency of work-related stressors or nurse burnout. In a correlational-descriptive study to identify stressors associated with burnout in critical care nurses and nurses in other specialties, Cronin-Stubbs found that intensity or perceived impact rather than frequency of job stressors contributes to burnout. For example, the death of one patient in critical care may affect nurses more adversely than the daily pressures of caring for acutely ill patients. Also, significant life events in the presence of high job stress contribute to burnout. The study recommends that critical care nurses control the number and impact of stressors experienced at one time and balance negative with positive changes in their personal and occupational lives. As Cronin-Stubbs notes, "Critical care nurses encountered frequent and intense occupational stressors. Alternating periods of intensity with patients or activities that are less emotionally demanding, such as spending time alone, or decreasing the number of longterm, multi-traumatic patient/nurse relationships per case load, may reduce stress".

J. L. Stehle conducted a literature review on critical care nursing stress. Noting that studies from 1969 to 1972 portrayed critical care units as environments fraught with potential stress for nurses, Stehle questioned: "Where did the realization of critical care stress begin. How does it compare with other nursing stress. and, How active have nurses been in identifying, investigating and alleviating stresses specific to critical care."

Stehle found that nursing in general was described as stressful before critical care nursing was associated with stress. A 1960 study identified tensions of hospital nursing as patient suffering and death, heavy demands, frightening tasks, and disturbing relationships with patients. In 1965, P. A. Holsclaw identified the following areas of high emotional risk in nursing: the inability to restore patients to well-being and feelings of loss for patients with, for example, kidney transplantation, surgical risk, severe disability, rehabilitation problems, psychiatric difficulties, terminal illness, and critical illness. As early as 1965, writers alerted nursing, medicine, and other professions to the dangers inherent in the "intensively concentrated hospital environment".

The early studies and articles all viewed stress as a negative factor, but few authors agreed on a definition of the term "stress." These articles attempted to emphasize the presence of stress in critical care and to identify antecedents to actual stress. Koumans reported that the two most stressful aspects of one ICU were rapid turnover of staff through rotation and intensity of emotion in interpersonal interaction. Strauss reported the following stress antecedents for ICU nurses: complicated machinery, a narrow patient care focus, great responsibility, conflicts with the administration, and a crisis atmosphere. Nurse satisfactions related to intimacy, morale, and challenge were also reported. Vreeland and Ellis noted that patients' physical and psychological conditions were deemed the most stressful aspect of ICU work by nurses themselves. Tensions were described as direct stresses involving patient care and indirect stresses involving environmental phenomena. Vreeland and Ellis made a significant observation about the paradoxical nature of the ICU nurse's situation: warmth and sympathy are expected together with objectivity and assertiveness.

Later stress studies provided schemes for categorizing critical care stresses. C. B. Bilodeau categorized external stressors into five groups: patients, staff, environment, patients' families, and others. Hay and Oken identified twelve groupings of stressors: "heavy lifting, cardiac research, unpredictable scheduling, heavy responsibilities, patient anxiety, hectic pace, annoyance by patients' families, severity of patients' illness, lack of ample time off, insecurity, patient personalities, and nurse-nurse conflicts." The categories of stresses in a neonatal ICU reported by M. S. Jacobson included nurse-physician problems, understaffing, heavy work load, sudden death or relapse of an infant, personal insecurity, and the shock of sight and smells.

Most of the studies reviewed by Stehle reflect both the human response of the nurse to the patient crisis and the nurse's reaction to the structural components of the occupational setting or work relationships. Notably, most of these studies were conducted when ICU environments and patient crises were simpler and less technical than they have become since the early 1970s. The increasing use of ventilators for patient support, organ transplants, cardiac surgery, and the availability of advanced trauma care have increased both the complexity and the ethical dilemmas that health care personnel and consumers must confront. The stresses of these latter factors remain unassessed. A 1982 appraisal of stress and ICU nursing by E. H. Friedman supports his earlier observations that a sense of mastery and self-confidence can serve as an antidote to stress. According to Friedman, a 1980 survey of stress in 1,800 ICU nurses conducted by J. T. Bailey, D. Walker, and N. Madsen indicated almost complete agreement that the following factors in the ICU caused the most stress: conflict with other health care providers, inadequate staffing patterns, lack of support in dealing with death and dying, inadequate work space and other inefficient factors in the physical work environment, and unresponsive nursing leadership. Interpersonal relationships are the greatest source of ICU job stres. As Friedman notes, most ICU stress studies indicate that interpersonal relationships in patient care are reported by nurses both as sources of stress and as sources of satisfaction. Further, environmental demands that are appraised by one ICU nurse as stressful may be appraised by another nurse as satisfying or challenging. Friedman proposes assertiveness training for ICU nurses to increase "vigor and self-confidence." He notes that "exposure to high stress with adequate support and skill does not increase the risk of mental and physical illness".

Rudlof Moos has proposed a model for understanding the crisis of physical illness. Background and personal factors, illnessrelated factors, and physical and social environmental factors influence cognitive appraisal (the perceived meaning of illness), which influences adaptive tasks and coping skills. Moos proposes that the outcome of the crisis is determined by this process. He notes that the stresses faced by health care staff stem both from the nature of the tasks they perform and the way in which hospitals are organized. Especially in ICUs, the excessive workload and understaffing, fast pace and overstimulation, the lack of time for reflection and minimal control over the pace and organization of daily activities, repetitive activities such as taking vital signs every fifteen minutes, the alertness required to handle complex machines and procedures, and the frequent emergencies are significant stresses for nursing staff.

Other demands and stressors for critical care nurses result from patient care. As Moos notes, "the threat and incessant reality of death, the need to continue full nursing care and involvement with patients with little hope for survival or who are in an unconscious limbo where life is maintained only by machines, forces nurse to confront their feelings about death on a daily basis'". Other sources of stress for ICU nurses stem from the interpersonal aspects of the nurse's role as mediator and coordinator of the many individuals who come into an ICU each day. These persons include distraught families, frightened patients, and physicians who may cope with their own distress by diverting anger to nurses or by abdicating their responsibility and leaving the nurse to communicate medical issues to the patient's family. Moos notes that when doctors use distancing as their main coping strategy they shift responsibility for the patient's emotional health to the nurses.

As Moos describes, nurses may cope with stress in various ways. The phenomenon of burnout has been discussed previously. Moos notes that health professionals can avoid this "'caregiver's plight'" by effectively coping with the stressors they experience. Individual coping strategies include constructively using denial (ignoring permanent disfigurement and focusing on a patient's assets), achieving satisfaction from the challenge of a difficult job, using humor, accepting one's own feelings (depression or anger) as natural human reactions, and finding peer support. Organizations can enhance stress reduction by providing support groups and stress reduction resources. Further, hospital policies and structures can be altered to reduce stress. Staffing patterns in critical care can be made more flexible to allow for maximal time off, rest, and periods of temporarily rotating out of high-stress aress.

Increasing numbers of health care workers recognize the positive effects of exercise and relaxation and are incorporating these behaviors into their lifestyle patterns. Effective communication, assertiveness training and limit setting for and by nurses, and self-care activities can also be helpful. Nurses and physicians have become increasingly aware of the positive effects of touch, verbal comfort, relaxation techniques, and music in patient care. The outcomes for patients and staff have been the focus of recent studies. Positive physiologic and psychologic measures, including lowered blood pressure, anxiety, and pain, have been reported after the use of therapeutic touch.

New technology imposes both benefits and problems on critical care nurses. Sophisticated computerized systems provide nurses with highly accurate and precise physiologic measurements, giving a timely picture of the patient's status and facilitating rapid intervention if complications develop. Nurses may receive automatic assessments of chest drainage, urine output, and hemodynamic measures every two minutes. Some computer systems can be programmed to administer blood, fluids, or drugs to patients in small increments based on the computer's frequent assessment of measures of volume loss or changes in blood pressure. Some new technologies replace very invasive, high-risk techniques with less costly and problematic ones. Automation can help the nurse accomplish timely interventions, because critical changes in patient status may occur very quickly and require rapid and accurate decision making.

But technology also has hazards. Patient injury as a consequence of treatment, termed iatrogenic injury, has become a possibility as a result of invasive monitoring techniques. Such risks become even more likely in an era of nursing shortage and entry of inexperienced personnel. In a five-year study N. S. Abramson found that 25 percent of iatrogenic incidents occurred during July and August, a season typically associated with the presence of new interns, residents, nurses, and other health care personnel. V. Sinclair notes that the constant introduction of new technology into critical care units compounds the problem of undertrained personnel. Sinclair does not consider another complicating factor that contributes to the hazard of new equipment – the lack of uniformity in the equipment of the new technologies. Free market competition by companies and cost containment efforts by hospitals add to the constant change in critical care settings.

The highly technical ICU environment has received the attention of writers concerned with the impact of technology on nursing practice. P. A. DeVisser notes that the coordination inherent in providing twenty-four-hour nursing at the bedside can reduce the various problems of fragmentation of care, including contradicting therapies prescribed by multiple members of the health team. Further, the nurse can assess subtle subjective changes in a patient's level of consciousness, which technology cannot do. Finally, the nurse must take the continuous data both from technology and from human observation, and then assess and act on them appropriately.

As Susan Blackburn observes, in her examination of the neonatal ICU as a high-risk environment, concerns related to resource allocation, appropriate intervention, and treatment decisions are always present in these areas. The application of advanced technology that helps more infants survive is costly in material and human terms. Caretakers must deal with the constant bombardment of stimuli, the demands to perform very highly technical tasks, and the constant moral and ethical issues related to the use of extraordinary technology. Consumers must confront the cost of salvaging smaller and smaller infants in terms of equipment, personnel training, and the cost of long-term care of infants who may have physical, mental, and emotional handicaps as a result of surviving treatment. The developmental, financial, and emotional costs to families and to the infants as they grow have yet to be fully discerned, as does the impact of a high-stress environment so early in life on infants who survive.

Technology, especially computers, influences nursing care. Loretta Birckhead has found that computer operation and paperwork require more of the nurse's time than combined patient care areas of teaching and counseling, talking with family, nursing care planning, and socialization with the patient. Only three areas — basic nursing care, special treatments, and consultation — required more nursing time than the computer. Birckhead raises the following concerns that she believes nursing must consider as technology increasingly becomes a part of patient care. As expensive equipment is introduced into patient care areas questions of corporate profit versus patient interests may arise. Guidelines for raising questions in these areas are unclear. Nursing, as yet, has not designed safeguards to protect its role with patients as new technology is introduced in patient care and accepted as if "it is an improvement on the old".

Doris Carnevali outlines responsibilities of nurses with regard to technology. The nurse must know patient phenomena that require the use of specific equipment, know expected outcomes as patient and machines interact, know how to operate machines safely, and recognize patient cries that indicate effective or ineffective uses of equipment. Carnevali does not deal with the morality of equipment use. She accepts the "goal" of technology and advises nurses to adapt themselves to the equipment.

In her study of the relationship between nurses' empathy and technology, J. Howard Brunt lists stress, burnout, dehumanization, and fragmentation as adverse effects of technology. Brunt believes that nursing care is based on providing a therapeutic interpersonal relationship with empathy as a primary ingredient. Because technological environments are fraught with obstacles to interpersonal openness and communication, the effect of nurses' empathy, especially in ICUs, is an important issue. In Brunt's comparison of empathy responses of nurses from four clinical units as varied as rehabilitation and surgical ICU, the surgical nurses perceived that they worked in a more technical unit than the other nurses, but all nurses scored very low on an empathy scale. Brunt notes that her results deviate from those of other investigators, where nurses were found to score average to high in empathy, but recommends that nurses should be taught content on empathy in nursing schools and in continuing education offerings.

Policy decisions regarding resource allocation for heroic medicine versus prevention continue to be debated in state arenas. Perhaps the most recent widely publicized controversy surrounding advances in medical technology is the artificial heart debate. Since 1982, when Barney Clark received the "Jarvik-7" artificial heart, the artificial heart has been implanted in four other persons. The machines were crude, quality of life for all these patients was very poor, and all the patients have died. In addition, other mechanical devices that boost the heart (left ventricular assist devices) and are used to support patients awaiting heart transplant are not without their own high risk of complications. Taken together, these machines bring limited benefit to very few at very great cost.

The media attention focused on the use of the "Jarvik-7" seems to imply that the use of artificial organs is somehow new. In fact, the first artificial organ, the kidney dialysis machine, is now forty-six years old. Other artificial devices and drugs that support natural organic or sensory functions include items as varied as dentures, eye glasses, hearing aids, artificial limbs, and insulin, estrogen, testosterone, or thyroid hormone. Artificial organs are significant in the context of this discussion because of the philosophical issues they raise – prevention versus treatment, resource allocation, and public policy decisions about funding for prevention, research, and treatment programs. Questions of scarce resources for a few versus prevention or care for many remain active public health and policy issues.

Problems related to overdependence on technology include a decline in clinical assessment skills; machine error; inability to detect errors, "trouble-shoot," or repair faulty equipment; and the legal implications of contradictory computer data. Increased liability, increased stress, and depersonalized care have been outcomes of a highly technical environment. As Ellen Rudy and Donna Lee Bertram point out, in addressing the trends in biomedical technology toward new knowledge, new technology, and increased costs, sophisticated machines have begun to assume many functions formerly controlled by human workers because machines can be programmed to perform more accurately. Technology also presents copious amounts of data, more than can be fully interpreted. The crux of the challenges of efficacy and efficiency is testing new ideas and discarding old methods that no longer apply. In their discussion, however, Rudy and Bertram present technology as a panacea. They do not consider the realities and constraints of rapid change, the economics of cost containment, and the complex demands of the critical care environment. The critical care unit was not developed as a controlled laboratory for scientific testing of new technologies. The realities and values of that setting are not a controlled technological environment.

Sallie Tisdale addresses the complexities and subtleties of this critical care environment in a poetic reflection:

They want help, these people. So do I. We need help in answering certain fundamental questions. Help in asking the question in the first place. Our need goes far beyond economic hand-wringing or ethics committees. It demands an acknowledgement of the surreal reality of the sick, and of the maelstrom in which health professionals stagger. The fecundity of the technology, the sheer weight of the machinery cause us to lament, and yet the surf catches us and sweeps us out to sea. We never think to swim back – we've forgotten how to swim.

Dolores M. Garlo also discusses the legal dimensions of contemporary critical care nursing practice. She points out that the scope of critical care nursing practice has generated particular areas of liability. These areas of responsibility often overlap with physician tasks or with former physician tasks. Areas of potential liability include informed consent, patient care activities and the use of technological devices, decisions regarding life-sustaining treatment, and patient protection. The development of critical care nursing paralleled developments in medicine. The evolution of nursing, of which critical care was a part, has broadened the scope of nursing responsibility. This evolution has been judicially recognized, and nurses have assumed increasing liability for malpractice as well as simple negligence.

Garlo identifies three distinct phases in the development of nursing and the evolution of legal regulation. Her first phase begins in the 1800s, when nursing was voluntary and no specific training or licensing was required. During this phase, the first nursing schools in the United States, based on the "Nightingale model" opened in 1873 in New York, Connecticut, and Massachusetts. Nursing schools increased in number during the early 1900s, and hospitals used nursing students, rather than graduates, as a cheap source of labor. In fact, nurses were not employed in hospitals in any numbers until the 1930s and later, at the onset of World War II. The first professional nursing organizations were organized in the early 1900s, and members lobbied for registration or state control to provide quality standards for patient care.

The scope of nursing practice was first defined in terms of specific functions that the nurse was allowed to perform. Since physician practice had been previously defined, the focus of defining nursing practice centered on differentiating it from the practice of physicians. Labor issues came to the forefront during this period. The hospital lobby eclipsed both the drive for increased economic benefits for nurses and the rights of nurses to bargain collectively.

By the 1950s, nursing practice had progressed beyond the existing nurse practice acts. Many nurses were already active in the acts of observation, data collection, and decision making regarding methods of patient care. Although the physician continued to prescribe treatment, the nurse determined the most appropriate way to implement care for a particular patient. Although the Nurses' Association proposed a model definition of nursing to reflect current practice, independent judgment remained legally unrecognized.

The third phase of legal history in nursing occurred in the mid- 1960s, with a shift toward medical specialization.

The locality rule, first established in 1880, was discarded in 1968 by the same court that created it. A national standard of care for a specialty practice was imposed. Under the locality standard, a patient with chest pain in a rural area received the best care that the small hospital or physician could deliver. With the introduction of a national standard, the specialty standards of cardiology were imposed in all circumstances and settings. Health care was becoming a huge industry, and hospitals grew as employers and as businesses as a consequence of the enlarging insurance industry. Furthermore, the increase in medical specialization decreased the numbers of general practitioners and created a gap in primary care. Nursing responded to this crisis by placing practitioners in clinic settings. These nurses were, in fact, often diagnosing and treating patients in direct violation of nurse practice acts.

Medical specialization also had begun to impact hospital care, and nursing specialization in hospitals paralleled the development of medical specialties. The development of coronary care units and intensive care units placed hospital nurses in the same violation of practice acts as the nurses in primary care, including making diagnoses and differentiating signs and systems for the purpose of initiating treatment. Many state nursing and medical associations attempted to resolve this dilemma, but laws in some states continued to prohibit nurses from diagnosing or initiating treatment in any circumstances, despite long-standing acceptance of this reality by both medicine and nursing.

As Garlo notes, nursing throughout its development has consistently expanded its role into the domain traditionally defined as medicine as a result of unionization pressures, improved curricula in schools of nursing, and rapid advances in medical knowledge and technology. Further, nurses in these expanded roles provide services that are more cost effective than are some services provided by physicians. With consensus of approval by medicine and nursing, general duty nurses "elicit and record health histories; interpret selected laboratory findings; make diagnoses in certain situations; choose, initiate, and modify selected therapies in selected situations; provide emergency treatments; and make prospective decisions regarding treatment in collaboration with physicians". Critical care nurses routinely perform all these tasks formerly initiated only by physicians. Garlo argues that this redefinition in roles warrants legal recognition.

This redefinition process actually took place in Georgia, following a ruling in early 1988 by State Attorney General Bowers that only physicians could diagnose and treat patients. The law had been passed in an effort to keep optometrists from operating with lasers, decreeing that only physicians, veterinarians, dentists, and podiatrists could "perform any surgery, operation, or invasive procedure" using any mechanical means to cut or alter either human or animal tissue. The law in effect made many routine nursing tasks, such as giving an injection, initiating an intravenous line, or wound care, illegal. The law threw the entire health care community into confusion, and was finally ruled unconstitutional by the Georgia Supreme Court in its 1992 session.

The earliest critical care units were postoperative recovery rooms. As described by Florence Nightingale in 1859"it is not uncommon, in small country hospitals to have a recess or small room leading from the operating theater in which the patients remain until they have recovered, or at least recovered from the immediate effect of the operation". The concept of grouping very ill patients close to the nurse for observation and care is often attributed to Nightingale. The development of critical care units coincided with developments in medical technology and medical specialization. Trauma care during World War II and the Korean and Vietnam wars refined medical and nursing skills. Advances in mechanical ventilation, notably the iron lung, and parallel developments in immunology and microbiology revolutionized treatment and prevention of poliomyelitis (polio). Soon, concepts that had been successful in the treatment of respiratory effects of polio were applied to the treatment of patients with varied pulmonary diseases, such as asthma, acute pulmonary edema, and respiratory failure. A group of life-support techniques became refined and generally available in the 1960s. These techniques included prolonged endotracheal intubation and mechanical ventilation, closed chest cardiac massage and defibrillation, continuous electrocardiographic monitoring, electrical and drug reversal of cardiac arrhythmias and electrical pacemaking, bedside cardiac catheterization with flow-directed catheters, analysis of respiratory gases in arterial and mixed venous blood, intra-aortic balloon counterpulsation, hemodialysis, and hemodynamic monitoring. Recovery rooms were soon followed by respiratory, coronary, neurosurgical, renal dialysis, and cardiac surgical care units.

The nursing shortage following World War II was another factor that contributed to the development of intensive care units. Prior to the emergence of the intensive care unit, all hospital patients were cared for on the general ward, in rooms with one, two, or more beds. Open wards with ten to twenty beds were common, especially in public and military hospitals or in sections of private hospitals designated for indigent care. The sickest patients would be moved closest to the nurses' station or would be cared for by a private duty nurse. According to Barbara Melosh, hospital administrators saw the early intensive care units (ICUs) as a solution to staffing problems and as a model of efficiency. Fewer nurses could care for more patients, private duty nurses would become obsolete, and highly skilled workers and equipment would be concentrated in one area. Managerial expectations were short-sighted, however. Staffing requirements both in the ICU and in the wards increased as medical intervention and treatment became more complex and sophisticated. The ICU development occurred as much in response to an enlarging capacity for expert care as for economic reasons. As Charles Rosenberg notes, "one can hardly understand the evolution of the hospital without some understanding of the power of ideas, of the allure of innovation, of the promised amelioration of painful and incapacitating symptoms, through an increasingly effective hospital-based technology."

The intensive care units of the early 1950s were similar in a number of features, although they developed independently in different parts of the country. Many were located in small quarters that had been hastily converted to ICU care. Although both medical and surgical patients were admitted to the units, surgical patients were in the great majority. In fact, many units were planned to care for patients having specialized thoracic or cardiac surgery and neurosurgery. The ICUs were open wards, with beds separated by a screen or curtain, with equipment crowding the cramped floor space. Visiting privileges were limited or absent. Staff learned on the job and traditional nursing skills provided the foundation for care.

The ICU concept was adopted by hospitals very quickly and changes in physical design and total environment were incorporated as ICUs became increasingly common. Many units opened at about this time in many places; in fact, a number of hospitals claim the "first" ICU or CCU. Of these, the Rhode Island Hospital, which in 1955 opened the first ICU in a working space that was specifically designed for ICU use, provides an appropriate case for examining the environmental changes that were incorporated in the early ICUs. The Rhode Island Hospital unit was specialized in that it only admitted surgical patients. It was larger than the first units, with twenty-eight beds organized into four working areas. Most of the patients were in private rooms, under direct visual surveillance of the nurse from the central nursing station. The private patient rooms had outside windows and had "piped in" oxygen and suction. Each unit had a blood pressure manometer on the wall. A physician house officer was present in the ICU at all times, and a room was provided as sleep space for this physician. Special charting procedures were developed, and registered nurses assumed more complex responsibilities, some of which had previously been performed only by physicians. Visiting privileges were liberalized and could be flexible at the discretion of the nurse.

The design features of the Rhode Island ICU continued to influence later ICUs. The physical design, especially private rooms with outside windows, was more considerate of the patient's psychological needs. The scope of nursing practice was broadened, moving into territory previously the prerogative of the physician. The unit design accommodated longer patient stays in the ICU. And greater specialization of nursing skills was fostered, rewarded, and ultimately required. There was evidence that the early ICU had the beginnings of a training program to prepare nurses for the special knowledge and skills required to work in such a complex unit, but little detail exists about this preparation.

As the environments of acute and psychiatric hospitals have gained the attention of environmental psychologists, research has emerged in three major areas. The first studies that examined the effects of the physical layout of hospital space on social interaction concentrated on balancing patients' needs for social contact and privacy. From these studies have come current cubic and circular hospital designs. Many of the designs that facilitate nursing observation interfere with patient privacy. Recommendations from these types of studies have resulted in such details as private/semiprivate rooms, lounge areas for visitors and nursing staff, patient bathrooms designed with privacy in mind, and play rooms for children and adolescent patients.

Second, studies have focused on the stressors in the environment, especially levels of stimulation for patients and staff. Studies have examined the effects of varied levels of information and sensory input on patients and staff. The impact of stress on patients, families, and nurses in critical care settings has been discussed previously. The stress studies also generated data that have been used to alter environmental stimuli. Lighting, noise, and noxious stimuli have been altered in the design of ICUs. Muted lighting, soft music, clocks, color, doors that close, calendars, windows, conditions that enhance sleep, and the presence of personal posses sions are just a few examples of this phenomenon. Similarly, attention has been directed to monitoring information overload for patients in high stress areas so that appropriate information may be received and incorporated effectively.

Finally, studies have dealt with the needs and abilities of patients to exact personal control over information access and the details of the hospital experience. Hospital care has shown steady trends toward participatory styles of care and patients' rights. In fact, studies indicate that patients who exert choice and control experience better morale and improved health status.

The conflicts experienced by patients in attempting to deal with hospital environments are perhaps best expressed by Norman Cousins in describing his recovery from a heart attack. He cites the following stressors: lack of respect for basic sanitation, the high risk of exposure to infectious agents, and the overly extensive use of x-ray and other technical equipment. Admitted to an ICU, Cousins was bemused by the "circular paradox to intensive care units...where patients are provided with better electronic aids than ever before for dealing with emergencies that are often intensified because they communicate a sense of imminent disaster". Concluding that "a hospital is no place for a person who is seriously ill." Cousins left the hospital and entered a hotel room for peace and quiet at about one-third the cost.

Nurses have a profound impact in shaping the hospital environment for patients. As Rosenberg notes in his study of the rise of the hospital industry, patients and families have come increasingly to depend on strangers to care for loved ones in illness and death: "Perhaps the most important single element in reshaping the day-to-day texture of hospital life was the professionalization of nursing. In 1800, as today, nurses were the most important single factor determining ward and room environment. Nursing, like professional hospital administration and changed modes of hospital financing has played a key role in shaping the modern hospital".

As Mary Anne Noble notes, the environment of patients has always been the nurse's concern. Nurses "control" the patient's environment by shaping, changing, developing, creating, and maintaining various details. Noble believes that the nurse perceives the fluctuations of daily routines and their effects on patients because of caring for patients around the clock. The nurse may create a therapeutic milieu or may manipulate factors in the environment to a therapeutic outcome. Thus, the environment of patients has become the special concern of nursing.

Rudolf Moos elaborates on specific measures that nurses and other hospital staff can employ to humanize the hospital environment. These efforts include allowing patients to participate in their own care and to control as many details of care as possible, placing patients in private rooms or cubicles for privacy, turning down the lights at night, scheduling procedures so patients can have free time, keeping monitors out of patients' rooms, and providing a more normal and cheerful environment through the use of color on walls, linens, and curtains. Further, a sense of personal identity can be promoted by allowing patients adequate space, privacy, and personal belongings. Moos recommends attention to both physical and social design so that the beneficial impact of hospital settings may be enhanced.

In the early 1960s, almost a third of patients admitted to a hospital after a heart attack died. Death occurred not from the occlusion of the coronary artery but from the complications associated with it, particularly arrhythmias that interrupted normal electrical conduction, causing cardiac arrest and circulatory failure as a consequence of the failing heart. The technological advances of cardiac monitoring, cardiopulmonary resuscitation, defibrillation, cardioversion, and hemodynamic, biochemical, and metabolic monitoring provided mechanisms of immediate treatment for lethal arrhythmias, cardiac arrest, ventricular fibrillation, and primary pump failure. Principles from these technological advances formed the basis of the coronary care unit. In these units the combined action of special observational techniques, skilled nursing, and specialized medical care prevented deaths from complication of AMI by detecting and immediately treating complications. The earliest units were established in 1962 and 1963 in Toronto; Kansas City, Kansas; Philadelphia; and Melbourne and Sydney, Australia. The implementation of the coronary care unit spread rapidly, revolutionizing the care of the hospitalized patient and the practice of nursing in the hospital setting.

Coronary care units reduced mortality from acute myocardial infarction and improved the treatment of cardiac arrhythmias. These units became the prototype of intensive care limited to a medical specialty. Further, as treatment of primary problems improved survival, patients lived to experience failure of another physiologic system, or to experience iatrogenic problems acquired as a consequence of hospitalization or treatment.

Technology triggered the reality of multi-system instability or failure. For example, successful treatment of a heart attack might be accompanied by a drop in blood pressure, which could cause a stroke or kidney failure. Often, all systems could be supported with technology until the patient died of massive infection or bleeding, or suffered brain death.

The nurse in the coronary care unit rapidly became the major treatment modality. The nurse was skilled, could implement treatment, and was there twenty-four hours a day. The nurse made electrocardiographic observations, diagnosed the specific types of cardiac arrhythmias, and prescribed electrical and drug therapy, frequently in the absence of physician support. This delegation of major diagnostic, decision-making, and treatment activities by physicians to nurses represented something new. This role change, as we have seen, also placed the nurse in violation of most state nurse practice acts.

The trends in technology, role changes for nursing, and management of complex patients seen in the evolution of the recovery room and coronary care unit occurred in the cardiac surgical intensive care units as improved techniques of cardiac catheterization, extra-corporeal circulation (the heart-lung machine), prosthetic valves and grafts, coronary revascularization, and repair of congenital heart defects made open heart surgery on adults and children safe and effective. Later technologies in the 1970s, 1980s, and 1990s such as the artificial heart and the transplant of single and multiple donor organs, have continued the trends identified above.

The nursing literature in the early 1970s provides two cautionary responses to the intensive care unit phenomenon. Esther Lucille Brown reflected on the implications of the development of intensive care and raised two questions. The first concerned the cost of critical care – the presence of a heavily staffed ICU serving a few patients at the expense of "good care" or regular hospital services. The second dealt with the nature and scope of patient care in the ICUs themselves. The trend toward bringing highly competent staff and patients in close proximity to equipment neglected considerations of the physical environment, patient expectations and perceptions of care, the impact of the environment on nurses, nurse-physician relationships, and the role of the nurse in providing total care. Brown had, in 1948, articulated some of the issues that concerned nursing educators and practitioners as nurses began to assume a more highly skilled and technical role in patient care, especially in assuming tasks previously performed by physicians. Concern at that time was expressed about preparation, competence, and retention of those caretaking and comfort skills considered to be the art of nursing.

The second note of caution was voiced in 1972 by Julia Munch, the editor of a *"Symposium on Units for Special Care."* Munch offered the concern that special care not be reserved for the seriously ill patient in a coronary or intensive care unit, a burn unit, or a pulmonary unit to the detriment of the patient receiving intermediate, long-term, self, and home care. Munch made a plea that special care be defined as individualized care and that this care be delivered to all patients.

By mid-century the Nurses' Associations had become increasingly involved with legislative and bargaining issues, and perhaps less involved with clinical practice. Indeed, throughout its history, ANA seems to have been at variance with the views and interests of the practicing nurse. Consequently, clinical organizations grew rapidly and assumed many of the functions of the professional organization. The Association of Operating Room Nurses had been established in . The Association of Critical Care Nurses was incorporated in 1969. Its goals reflected the practice and education issues of concern to nurses in diverse critical care settings. The emergence of ACN paralleled the development of other clinical specialty organizations in nursing in areas such as orthopedics, neurosurgery, obstetrics, pediatrics, post-anesthesia care, and rehabilitation. The fragmentation that resulted has been partially resolved by a late 1970s consortium of clinical organizations with the ANA named the Nursing Organization Liaison Forum. This consortium promotes collaboration and communication between the diverse nursing groups.

Critical care nursing grew rapidly from its roots in the postoperative recovery room. The growth of technology and of medical specialization encouraged a parallel growth in the numbers and types of ICUs. The ICU prototype – a small unit with a mix of medical and surgical patients – can now only be found in the small community hospital. Coronary care units (CCUs), medical ICUs (MICUs), and surgical ICUs (SICUs) are standard in most community hospitals. In major teaching and medical centers, specialty ICUs of every type exist, including pediatric, renal, burn, respiratory, neurosurgical, heart surgery, and organ transplant ICUs, in addition to the CCU, MICU, and SICU. The trend toward highly specialized units continues. Furthermore, the newer ICUs reflect changes in focus from acute care to include trauma, rehabilitation, chronic, and long-term care. Patient stays in ICUs may range from several days to many months.

The nurse emerged as the major treatment modality in the evolving critical care unit. Nurses incorporated many roles, some that had been the purview of the physician and some that were new to both medicine and nursing. While many technical support occupations evolved in health care, nursing continued to incorporate the highly complex skills brought about by technology and specialization into the traditional caring role. Nursing assumed the responsibility for training nurses in critical care skills in the hospital rather than in the academic setting, although graduate education in critical care also developed as a way of preparing clinical nurse specialists, and critical care content began to be included in undergraduate curricula in some programs.

As critical care units became common in hospitals, concerns about the impact of high levels of stress on patients, families, and nurses began to emerge. The invasive and highly technical nature of the environment, the dehumanizing aspects of care, and the outcomes of the care itself – that is, recovery, death, or debility – were found to cause high levels of stress. Concerns continue to be raised about the influence of these pressures on attrition of nurses from hospital nursing.

The World has experienced a relative and actual nursing shortage since World War II. Various efforts to increase numbers of nurses through increased nurse training money have had a positive effect. However, increasing numbers of nurses are needed in complex critical care, and acute and non-acute ambulatory, chronic care, and home care, settings. Fewer women have entered nursing as a career because of increasing opportunities in other disciplines with greater opportunities for status and salary. This loss of nurses through attrition, whether from stress, low status or income, or increased opportunities elsewhere, merits study.

Little is known about the details of the experiences of the practicing nurse as critical care units evolved. Interviews with nurses involved in these settings reveal many insights into the roles of nurses, the scope of nursing practice, the stresses of the settings and the care, and the uniqueness of the nature of interactions of nurses and patients. In Margaret Mead's words, the nurse protects "those in danger...from illness, from strain, from shock, from sorrow, from grief". Interviews with critical care nurses may provide data about the precise nature of how they learned to do that as critical care settings evolved.

# Chapter 3

# The Critical Care Unit

## INTRODUCTION

Efforts have been made to humanize the critical care environment, but in fact, the critical care setting has become much more complex than that observed by Hay and Oken. But this scenario, because of its date, may well be representative of the experiences of the critical care nurses.

The physical structure and unique function of a critical care unit are as variable as the diverse hospitals. Many variables influence the characteristics of critical care units. The size and location of the hospital and the characteristics of the population served will influence whether the intensive care unit is small or large, in a rural or urban area, and whether the patients are young families or older, retired adults. The purpose of the hospital also influences the characteristics of the ICU. Small community hospitals have different patient populations than do large, tertiary medical centers. Some of the many criteria for admission include patient age and diagnosis, individual physician practices, community standards, formal criteria of hospital committees, bed availability, and nursing staff availability. Patients are admitted to critical care units for a variety of reasons. These include observation and surveillance of their primary medical condition or its complications, care and treatment of an acute illness or injury, postoperative care, either routine or complicated, and delivery of specialized technological monitoring or treatment.

The increasing size of the older adult population is another factor that influences the population of patients served in critical care units. Moreover, not only are patients living longer; they are surviving acute illness that would have been fatal in earlier years. Patients suffering from a chronic illness like diabetes now have extended lives as a result of successful management of their clinical health problems. These various population characteristics result in an older population of patients being treated in critical care units, who may have complicated health histories and repeated exacerbations of chronic health problems. Finally, the politics and economics of health care influence the populations seen in critical care units. Hospitals compete vigorously for those hospital services likely to be lucrative. These include, for example, emergency services and high-technology services such as cardiac procedures, organ transplant, and research therapies. Shifts in services provided by hospitals influence the characteristics of populations in critical care units. Hospitals that provide critical care for the indigent or uninsured, and those covered by various local and state welfare or Medicaid programs, are particularly influenced by the shifts in profitable services away from their hospitals. In fact, many of these hospitals have closed, leaving large populations of urban and rural poor unserved.

## TRENDS

Several trends influence all areas of health care, including critical care nursing. The escalating cost of health care has generated several outcomes that have had a broad impact on health care delivery. The prospective reimbursement system for hospital Medicare patients, introduced in 1983, and current managed care competition require cost containment measures and a redefinition of minimum standards of care for hospitalized patients. The patient care plan must reflect a strategy that best meets the patient's needs within time restrictions and limited resources. The goal of efficiency imposes shorter hospital stays for patients, restructuring of hospitals for economic survival, and attempts to quantify nursing care costs. Patients in hospitals are sicker, are being treated more expediently, and are being discharged before they are fully recovered from their illnesses. Home health care and ambulatory services are mushrooming in response to the need and the economic incentive.

A second trend in health care relates to the highly technical hospital environment. Rapidly changing technology imposes both knowledge requirements and a growing concern about the impersonality of the critical care environment. Nursing has responded to these issues by attempts at collaboration and communication in education and practice, innovative attempts at care planning through computerization, organized training and education plans for staff, and new roles and structures in nursing practice.

Nursing as a discipline is becoming inextricably bound to technology. Specialization in medical practice since the 1960s has imposed a national standard of medical and nursing care. Prior to that time, a physician might determine appropriate care for a heart attack patient. This care might be influenced by the region, the personal philosophy of the physician, and the resources of the community and hospital. The general practitioner in a small town might have a different standard than would the teaching hospital in a large city. This is less the case now than ever before. National medical board certification now determines obstetric or cardiac care in both urban and rural areas, and these standards are upheld legally for physicians, nurses, and hospitals.

Hospitals in small towns may have equipment and offer services once only seen in a medical center. Regional trauma and neonatal ICU networks illustrate this phenomenon. Third-party payers, including Medicare, impose a further standard for hospital care. Accreditation standards set by the Joint Commission on Accreditation of Healthcare Organizations also promote similarities rather than differences among hospitals. Critical care units have emerged as a common feature of hospitals in the 1990s. The consequences of technology for nursing practice include demands for education and training, the emergence of specialized clinical roles, creative and often expensive staffing patterns, salary incentive programs, concerns about attrition of expert staff, stress and job tension, and the stresses of ethical dilemmas arising in critical care settings.

Critical care nursing, now an expected part of hospital care in the 1990s, seems rooted in two distinct features. First, the magnitude of patient needs calls for twenty-four-hour nursing surveillance. The nature of this nurse-patient relationship has social, structural, institutional, and economic roots in the evolution of nursing. Private duty nursing and hospital staff nursing both contain elements of this model of nursing care. Second, the critical care unit has emerged as a geographic entity in hospitals, structuring patients and nurses together in response to medical and surgical specialization and increasing technology.

Critical care nursing may reflect other evolutionary changes in twentieth-century nursing. Nursing education has increasingly moved to collegiate settings, and changes in nursing practice include performance of comprehensive physical and psychosocial patient assessments. The emerging trend toward theoretically grounded practice and research has been steady. The practice of critical care nursing is increasingly complex and sophisticated. Further, the consequences of feminist ideology and labor practices in medicine and nursing practice in hospital settings are but two of the social trends that have influenced the larger society as well as nursing as a discipline. Questions about the distinctiveness of critical care nursing practice seem rooted both in past practice settings and in the unique interpersonal and technological environment of the contemporary critical care unit.

Several themes were consistent as nurses spoke about the evolution of the early intensive care units. Increasing specialization, knowledge, and technology precipitated a need for bringing together nurses who had specialized knowledge with patients. The private duty nurse-patient relationship seemed to be the model for this ICU planning, rather than the existence of equipment or technology. Many of the earlier ICUs opened even without cardiac monitors, now considered one of the most fundamental elements of ICU care. The nurse was the monitor in the early units, using traditional hands-on nursing skills, such as taking the pulse and temperature and providing constant surveillance and observation of patient condition and status. Both medicine and nursing were less complex then and often involved more touch and personal, hands-on ministrations and care, such as alcohol baths for persistent high fevers.

## CONTEMPORARY UNITS

As technology and specialized equipment emerged rapidly, the pace of change accelerated. This rapid change had several outcomes. Nurses were eager to learn new skills, but did not forfeit older methods. Nursing incorporated technical expertise into the traditional constant caretaking considered essential to nursing practice. Both medicine and nursing often experienced an over-reliance on technology that at times resulted in a diminished capacity for manual assessment.

Certainly, technology resulted in more data being available for both medicine and nursing. The nurse quickly became the expert in critical care. Since change was constant, there were few experts to teach and establish acceptable standards of practice. Nurses assumed new roles as clinical educators of nurses, patients, and often physicians, and as clinical experts who used clinical judgment to determine appropriate patient care. Nurses often set limits on patients, visitors, other nurses, and physicians in order to protect patients in the critical care unit. In reality, nurses always exercised judgment in hospitals to protect patients from harm or to provide better care. As the nurses in this study attest, in the days before the ICU the sickest patients were moved closest to the nurses' station so that the nurses could give them more continual nursing care. The physical space for the early ICUs was almost always adapted from areas not designed specifically for ICU care, often from space no longer needed because of technological advances. For example, steam rooms used for babies with croup or patients with pneumonia, which were made obsolete by the advent of antibiotics and the availability of humidified oxygen, were often converted to ICUs.

The changes in technology and the new nursing roles were always a surprise to nurses. Defibrillation of the heart, for example, was described as almost unbelievable. Implementation of new technology was similarly unclear and uncharted. The new coronary care unit described by Carla Olson opened waiting for formal admissions. The first patient had been admitted to a semiprivate room at 2:00 A.M. in the usual manner, and was admitted to the CCU only after he had a crisis. Nurses and physicians had good collaborative, working relationships in these specialized units. Both learned together that the technology and the care would increase patient survival.

The skill acquisition in adapting to new technology was additive. Nurses incorporated the new skills into traditional roles. Nurses in critical care have complex knowledge and skills, and they intervene based on that expertise. For example, nurses give drugs or defibrillate the heart based on their assessment of cardiac arrhythmias. Nurses also diagnose cardiac ischemia (low tissue oxygen level) from an electrocardiogram and notify the physicians, so that immediate intervention can prevent a heart attack or death. The combination of caring, skill, and continual presence was enhanced by a new aggressiveness in nursing practice in the critical care nurse. This aggressiveness in assessing and intervening with patients based on specialized knowledge was a new concept. It surprised and confounded many nurses and physicians.

The traditional nursing characteristics of caring, skill, and continual presence were augmented by a new aggressiveness as critical care settings became increasingly complex during the 1970s, 1980s, and 1990s. The nursing role was greatly amplified as nurses assumed responsibility for increasing numbers of technical skills. Technology influenced the practices of physicians and others in many medical and surgical specialties, for example, heart surgery in adults and children, renal dialysis, trauma care, and infectious disease. However, the technology at the bedside inevitably became the on-going responsibility of the nurse, often with very little anticipation or time for preparation. The various technologies, for example, ventilators, pulmonary artery catheters, cardiac, respiratory, and intracranial monitors, drug infusion pumps for almost any type of drug (narcotics, chemotherapeutics, vasopressors, vasoconstrictors, antiarrhythmics, metabolic support, and antibiotics), feeding tubes, and drainage devices (from the bladder, bowel, wounds, or chest cavity) – became routine patient care management strategies for the nurse at the bedside. Many support services emerged at this time to handle many of the technical aspects of one specialty, for example, renal dialysis technicians, anesthesia technicians, cardiopulmonary bypass technicians, and laboratory technicians. At this same time physician assistants emerged in a technical support role with physicians, and specialties in respiratory therapy and physical therapy began to develop. Nursing continued its traditional role of comprehensive patient care, perhaps in a medical or surgical specialty, while incorporating technology as it appeared at the bedside.

Providing adequate nurse staffing in hospitals, both in terms of quality of skill level and quantity, continued to be a problem. Two factors that influenced this issue were the insurance reimbursement systems by which hospitals receive operating costs and the organization of nursing services in hospital settings. Nurses are employed by hospitals. They do not bill patients for services. Nursing care, like housekeeping or dietary services, is included as a patient charge in the daily room rate. While recent efforts to "cost out" nursing services in hospitals and to obtain third-party reimbursement for nurses in independent roles have had some success with several insurance carriers and in several states, these cases remain in the minority. Many of the nurses interviewed identified inadequate staffing as a major stressor in critical care settings. These perceptions are consistent with the findings in the studies of nursing stress. Nurses generally identified hospital and nursing administrations as unresponsive to the highly stressful problems of understaffing or inflexible scheduling. Administrative reluctance to provide incentives to retain nurses, to increase nurse staffing, or to close hospital beds if necessary to provide safe nurse-patient ratios have often resulted in attrition of nurses from staff nurse positions in hospitals.

Nurses continued to value their personal involvement with patients and their families, even as the demand for increasingly complex skill acquisition increased. Nurses described the conflicts inherent in these interactions. The primary motivation for patient involvement for the nurses interviewed seemed to be making a difference in the lives of patients in crisis. Nurses were willing to assume responsibility for very intense commitment to patients and families, but nurses acknowledged great frustration when patients were caught up in crises of indecision about the use of technology. Nurses described situations where the existence of technology dictated its use. Margie Goodrum, for example, stated, "Our ability to do things has far outstripped our ability to decide when it is appropriate to do it."

Nurses embraced the technology and became proficient in it. Indeed, the nurse became the major treatment modality at the bedside. However, nursing incorporated that skill level into traditional roles. While nurses learned to generate and use the increased amounts of data available for patient care and appreciated the positive outcomes for patients, many conflicts emerged in the care setting as a result of high technology. Decision-making about the uses of technology and the increased data that were available remains a problem at many levels. Time is compressed with many new technologies. Patients, nurses, and physicians once had weeks or, at least, days to incorporate data and change, to teach, learn, and prepare for a procedure or technique. At present decisions often have to be made instantaneously. Technology is relentless and demanding. Carla Olson said, "Well, we are always playing catch-up. There is something new all the time and everything you hear of can either be a joke or the next most wonderful thing."

Finally, when technology is backed by faulty decision making, the nurses viewed it as causing inhumanity and unnecessary suffering. While critical care nurses are not alone in dealing with these conflicts, the continual presence of nurses at the bedside and their particular combination of caring and skill make the model of critical care nursing unique.

# Chapter 4

# The Science of Critical Care Nursing

## INTRODUCTION

The practicing nurse is almost invisible in the nursing literature. Case studies appear from time to time that reflect the intimacy of the nursepatient relationship. These often relate the extraordinary experiences of nurses with, for example, dying patients, patients waiting for transplant, or children with leukemia. While the views of nursing's practice, education, and labor management leaders are well known, the evaluation of clinical practice has received less attention. For example, the literature may describe appropriate clinical management of a patient having heart surgery, but reveal nothing about the personal experiences of the nurses and patients during the actual caretaking. The stories of physicians and their patients have been more often told. The writings of Lewis Thomas and William Carlos Williams provide many examples of the range of human emotions and experiences in the medical care of patients.

The critical care nurses speaks openly and often passionately about their beliefs and commitments about nursing and the rewards and frustrations of patient care. Many factors contribute to the nurses' perceptions about themselves and their practice. Several of these that have particular impact on the practice setting were selected for discussion: the roles that nurses assume; the values that permeate nursing education and practice; the accepted model of decision making in nursing; the ways that nursing has been defined by nursing leaders and others (because of the influence these definitions have on the formation of a professional self-image); and, finally, a research study examining clinical nursing practice from the perspective of practicing nurses.

Various disciplines have described the role of the nurse in critical care settings in relation to the medical, nursing, administrative, legal, historical, ethical, and even architectural dimensions of critical care. The nurse has been described as coordinator of patient care, collaborator with physicians and all other health team members, and promoter of activities to help the patient regain or maintain health. Nursing functions in critical care have been defined by legal experts as including "interpretive and anticipatory functions of the nurse involving decision making and action with regard to a patient in biophysical and/or psychological crisis, close monitoring of patients in lifethreatening situations...and rendering of life supporting treatment to patients who could not otherwise monitor the functional mechanisms underlying the life processes. The nurse must focus time and attention on mechanical aspects of treatment, anticipate subtle changes in patient status, and make quick decisions in emergency situations".

## NURSING PROCESS

Nursing roles have been described in a variety of contexts, but generally five roles are highlighted: practitioner, educator, consultant, researcher, and manager. Nurses also have been described as coordinators of care and as change agents. These roles have been consistent in the literature since the 1950s, regardless of the actual job title or setting.

Several concepts and values that have persisted in nursing education, nursing practice, and the nursing literature provide a conceptual framework for nursing practice. Patients are human beings with worth, dignity, and basic human needs that must be met. When these needs are not met, health problems or crises occur that require intervention by another person until the individual can resume responsibility for him- or herself. The patient has a right to quality health and nursing care delivered with concern, compassion, and competence. Increasingly, competent acute care or illness care is seen as a partial step toward wellness, prevention, and restoration. The therapeutic nurse-patient relationship is seen as a tangible and valid mechanism for healing. All behavior is meaningful, and individuals cope with crisis in proportion to their perceptions and resources .

Nursing as a process is recognized by various legal, professional, and accrediting bodies. The *Standards of Clinical Nursing Practice* used nursing process as a framework as did the *Standards for Nursing Care of the Critically Ill* .

The legal definition of nursing in most states includes a reference to nursing process. Further, state boards of nursing require knowledge of nursing process for licensing by examination. The steps of the nursing process are derived from the scientific method. They include assessment (systematic collection of data relating to patients and their problems), problem identification (analysis and interpretation of data), planning (choice of solutions), implementation (putting the plan into action), and evaluation (assessing the effectiveness of the plan and changing the plan as indicated by current needs). Nursing process is also a standard required by the Joint Commission on Accreditation of Healthcare Organizations: "Individualized, goal-directed nursing care is provided to patients through the use of the nursing process" .

While nursing process became formalized as the appropriate model of decision making, other models have been proposed. The role of intuition and creative problem solving in nursing care was explored by Benner .

Implicitly, critical care nursing incorporates all the generally understood and accepted definitions and functions of nursing practice. The founder of modern nursing, Florence Nightingale, proposed the following definition in 1859. Nursing is "to have charge of the personal health of somebody...and what nursing has to do...is to put the patient in the best condition for nature to act upon him" .

Jane Van de Vrede was a nursing leader in the early twentieth century who was instrumental in setting practice and education standards in Georgia. While addressing the role of the public health nurse in 1921, when the focus of nursing was primarily private duty, public health, or Red Cross nursing, she proposed the following definition of nursing: "Prevention of illness and disability...is the unique function of the public health nurse, because of the acceptance of the nurse by the population, and the ability of the nurse to teach prevention...with the least presumptuousness and fear of being misunderstood. To this phase of health work, the nurse can make the greatest contribution" .

The anthropologist Margaret Mead, addressing a national nursing conference in 1956, made the following observation: "I have tried to identify this thing that everybody who is a nurse does, and how the service you give to our society could be phrased. It seems to me that you protect the vulnerable, that you protect all those who are or could be in danger, in any kind of danger – from illness, from strain, from shock, from fatigue, from sorrow, from grief; that every spot in this society where there are those who are in danger and who need continuous concern, this is the place where you might function" . This definition seems an almost prophetic vision of the roles and relationships that exist between critical care nurses and very ill, dependent patients in the highly technical, rapidly changing contemporary critical care unit. Never, in the history of modern nursing, have patients been so vulnerable, so much in danger and in need of continuous concern.

Virginia Henderson, a nursing leader and educator, first proposed her definition of nursing in the 1940s. This widely accepted definition likely influenced the self-concept of generations of nurses to the present. "Nursing is...assisting the individual, sick or well, in the performance of those activities contributing to health or its recovery (or to a peaceful death) that he would perform unaided if he had the necessary strength, will, or knowledge. And to do this in such a way as to help him gain independence as rapidly as possible". She updated this definition in 1985: "The unique function of the nurse is to do for others what they would do for themselves if they had the strength, the will and the knowledge; and to do it in such a way that the recipient of the service acquires independence as soon as possible or an ability to cope with a health handicap, or to die with dignity when death is inevitable" . The subtle differences between the definitions reflect language changes, but also an assumption that nurses assist patients with activities related to self-care and coping with the outcomes of illness. The change may indicate areas of evolution and maturity in nursing and in Henderson herself during those years.

Georgia's Nurse Practice Act (USA)gives the following definition:

Practice of nursing as a registered professional nurse means the performance for compensation of any act in the observation, care and counsel of the ill, injured, or infirm; and in the promotion and maintenance of health with individuals, groups, or both throughout the lifespan. It requires substantial knowledge of the humanities, natural sciences, social sciences, and nursing theory as a basis for assessment, nursing diagnosis, planning, intervention, and evaluation. It includes, but is not limited to, provision of nursing care; administration, supervision, evaluation, or any combination thereof, of nursing practice; teaching; counseling; the administration of medications and treatments, as prescribed by a physician practicing medicine in accordance with Article 2 of Chapter 34 of this title, or a dentist practicing dentistry in accordance with Chapter II of this title, or a podiatrist practicing podiatry in accordance with Chapter 35 of this title.

The Nurses' Associations proposed the following definition of nursing in 1980: "Nursing is the diagnosis and treatment of human responses to actual or potential health problems" In addressing the question "To what extent are popular definitions of nursing consistent with traditions and generally sanctioned social mission." Rosella Schloffeldt critiqued the ANA definition as ambiguous and lacking clear logic. She proposed, instead, the following: "Nursing is the appraisal and the enhancement of the health status, health assets, and health potential of human beings."

Definitions of nursing seem valuable to the extent that they direct values and attitudes or reflect them. The reflections of critical care nurses may forge new dimensions of self-appraisal. Patricia Benner conducted paired interviews with novice and expert nurses in order to "uncover the knowledge embedded in clinical nursing practice" . The interview data reveal the following domains of nursing practice: the helping role, the teaching-coaching function, diagnostic and monitoring functions, management of rapidly changing situations, administering and monitoring therapeutic interventions and regimes, monitoring and ensuring the quality of health care practices, and organizational and work role competencies. Benner's domains and the competencies for each domain are given here in order to form a framework for interpreting the interview material in this book and as a reference for the non-nurse reader to clarify the scope of nursing practice. These domains of nursing practice provide a clear descriptive framework for nursing practice and are consistent with the themes described by various critical care nurses.

Several themes predominated as critical care nurses spoke about nursing practice and their motivations, satisfactions, frustrations, and perceptions of their value. Almost universally, they expressed some type of commitment about self, nursing, and caretaking. Many spoke of nursing as a vocation and expressed a desire to make a difference in the lives and health outcomes of patients and their families. Even nurses who were more neutral about vocational commitments seemed heavily invested in nursing, patients, or the clinical situation. None of the nurses interviewed seemed indifferent, negative, or impersonal about the nurse-patient interaction. Nurses believed that they made a difference to patients through their competence in the actual care that was delivered. Especially in critical care settings, nurses made an impact through clinical management of the total patient situation. Nurses accomplished this through coordination, competence, expert clinical judgment, and advocacy. Expert clinical judgment and advocacy often involved anticipating subtle changes in patient status before they occurred, acting on them appropriately, monitoring medical management, and initiating action to obtain competent medical care. The nurses saw themselves as making the hospital system work for patients.

Nurses described a great deal of satisfaction from nurse-patient interaction, regardless of the setting. Nurses used the phrase "nurses take care of patients" often. And "the only reason patients need to be in the hospital is nursing care." One nurse described the challenge of "instant intimacy." Nurses and patients, although strangers, may bond quickly when brought together by the crisis of illness in a critical care environment. Nurses can often humanize this situation of crisis, chaos, illness, and life and death balances. Further, the process of investment of self seemed to humanize the interaction for both the nurse, the patients, and those family or friends close to them.

## Nurse-patient Interaction

The nurse-patient interaction in critical care settings was described in very powerful and passionate ways by critical care nurses. The nurse was described as a humanizing link for the patient and family that assisted them in managing a return to wellness or health, recovery, or death. Nurses believed that patients who were in crisis were especially vulnerable and in need of nursing intervention. The nurse made a difference to patients through competence, caring, and management of the total care situation. The concepts of advocacy and commitment were persistent as nurses described their interactions with patients and their families.

Nurses expressed a sense of commitment to the well-being of patients. This was described as a vocation by many and was seen as quite satisfying. The value of making a difference in the lives of others was described as a privilege. Nurses were willing to use heart and mind to be what was needed for others at a given time, even at the cost of caring for themselves. This commitment was described as less a self-sacrifice than a finely developed set of skills that nurses were willing and able to use for the good of patients at a given time. Nurses, for example, performed many complex skills at one time in order to accomplish what a patient needed at a certain time — a painfree afternoon, a peaceful death, specific medical intervention.

Advocacy was described as a complex set of roles that nurses used to act for or in place of patients or their families. The nurse in a critical care setting was the first line of defense for a sick patient. Nurses were advocates through assessment of psychological and physiological parameters and intervention to get medical help. Advocacy also implied coordination, synthesis, and integration of the patient situation. Nurses were described as the fabric of the care that holds the patient together. Nurses are there twenty-four hours a day. Nurses protect patients from consequences of illness, from poor care by others, and from hospital mismanagement. Nurses also provide emotional support to patients and families. They make the hospital system work for patients. They see subtle changes before they are trends and seek out appropriate help. They also help mobilize the patient toward wellness by decreasing fear. Finally, advocacy involves interpreting the hospital system for patients and families.

Nurses especially valued the human link that they felt with dying patients or patients in intractable pain. Nurses often used creative methods or personal commitment to give hope and to be what a dying patient needed.

The stresses of trying to be so available to patients who might be chronically ill, acutely ill, or dying were described by many nurses. One nurse said, "There is a lot of pressure to assume that you are taking care of all of a person's needs." The satisfactions of the intimacy of nursing care seem to be achieved at a cost. The costs to nurses of this intense involvement with patients include the stresses of the hospital environment, the complex technology, and the potential for ethical conflict.

Technology as a stressor to critical care nurses was described earlier. It is but one of the perceived stressors. Others include the nature of the work itself, the hours, the demands, the perceived low self-esteem, and inadequate staffing patterns. Nurses perceived stress when factors intervened to prohibit them from making a difference in the lives of patients by providing the nursing care that the nurse believed was essential at the time. Nurses described a willingness to be a buffer between the patient and his or her crisis and pain and the rest of the environment. The nurse made the hospital system work for the patient, coordinated the various services for patient care, and balanced complex physiological parameters in order to stabilize a patient's status. The patient might be unconscious and dependent or awake and alert. In either case, the patient might be very sick and unstable and dependent on the nurse for critical decision making with regard to normal progress, detection, and treatment of complications, maintenance of complex drug administration, and acquisition of medical intervention if needed. Most of the time, the physician is only present at a patient's bedside if he or she has been called by the nurse. These behaviors were described as satisfying, but often also, as stressful.

Clearly, as the critical care unit evolved and became more specialized, complex, and highly technical, the nursing role changed in many significant ways. The nurse became the central feature and resource in the critical care unit — uniquely identifiable because of refined skills, a new aggressiveness in promoting patient advocacy, and emerging roles, which included coordinating the care of these very ill patients. Although the environment and many of the roles and skills were new, the critical care nurse incorporated them into the traditional roles and relationships that nurses have always had with patients. Thus, the tasks and responsibilities were additive. The consequences of these changes have in some cases increased the status and selfconcept of nurses and nursing and in others have precipitated almost a schizophrenic ambivalence about nursing practice. Certainly the experiences shared make visible many of the outcomes of the changes brought about by the evolving critical care environment.

As nursing shared in the positive outcomes of technology, it also shared in the lack of clarity in roles and relationships and the ethical dilemmas that increasingly occurred with highly technical interventions with patients. Nurses were a consistent presence with patients and families in these latter situations and had to forge new ways of coping with patients who did not do well.

One of the major outcomes of the critical care environment was the persistence of stress. Nurses described many aspects of critical care nursing as stressful. The work itself, often physically difficult, requires rapid, complex decision making and the outcomes have the potential of being lifethreatening. Knowing the seriousness of the tasks, many nurses described a fear of the unknown. Further, great demands are routinely placed on the nurse by patients, families, physicians, and nurse administrators. The assumption of these responsibilities by nurses in these situations is often not rewarded but expected as a part of the job. The critical care environment, shift work, low salaries and limited opportunities for advancement, low staffing and the liabilities associated with it, and dealing so constantly with both dying patients and the patients who represent medical failure are other factors discussed as stressful by critical care nurses.

One of the most frustrating and stressful situations described by many of the nurses involved the feelings associated with inflicting torture or ongoing painful treatments on patients for whom there was no hope of return to any quality of life. Similarly, seeing patients do well, or survive or increase their quality of life, was described as very rewarding and satisfying. Nurses often established meaningful reciprocal relationships with dying patients and their family members that generated personal satisfaction and a renewed energy to cope with further stressful patient situations. Even if patients died, or deteriorated, nurses felt satisfaction if they saw the impact of their own competency. Nurses felt rewarded if they made a difference and felt that what they had done with patients was worthwhile, even if the activities associated with nursing care were stressful.

Nurses reduced stress by finding ways of "making a difference" with patients through advocacy, touch, consistency in care, and creating an organization that worked for patients and staff. Flexibility in work schedules and part-time work for premium pay were other ways that nurses decreased stress and fatigue. Nurses used such things as diet, exercise, and a healthy social and family life to accomplish the same goals. The term "balance" was used by several nurses in describing successful coping strategies. The point was made that the stressors and the satisfaction in critical care are the same list. The challenge becomes a disaster when nurses lose whatever capacity they have for wholeness and balance.

# Chapter 5

# Resource Limits and Allocation in Critical Care

## INTRODUCTION

How much intensive care is necessary or justified. What kind of care should be available, and where and to whom should it be provided. How should society control the supply and use of intensive care. The widespread growth of intensive care, coupled with the heightened concern about health care costs, has focused attention on these and other related questions. The fact that these questions are being asked reflects a recognition of the competition between intensive care and other developing health care technologies for societal resources and other valued goods and services. Thus, the supply of intensive care is not unlimited. When such a valued resource is constrained, questions of how it should be distributed inevitably arise. Moreover, recent changes in the financing and delivery of health care are changing the historical influences on the development and provision of intensive care. This chapter will review the growth and current distribution of intensive care resources, as well as the possible causes and consequences of these patterns. Issues related to the allocation of societal resources to intensive care versus other health and welfare programs (that is, macroallocation) and the allocation of existing intensive care resources among patients (that is, microallocation) will also be discussed.

## PATTERNS

Intensive care has grown rapidly during the last two decades. Stimulated by the development of life-saving and monitoring tech niques requiring specialized personnel and equipment, intensive care units (ICUs) developed in a relatively uncontrolled fashion. Their spread was facilitated by the predominance of cost-reimbursement as a means of financing hospital care and the lack of hospital internal constraints on creating intensive care units. The approximately 80,000 intensive care beds currently available in hospitals are estimated to account for more than 15 percent of hospital charges. Almost 95 percent of acute care hospitals reportedly have intensive care beds.

The widespread availability of intensive care beds has made this type of care the current standard practice in many instances. Many patients who are at high risk for experiencing a complication requiring prompt treatment are now admitted to intensive care for monitoring. Intensive care is now considered routine following many complicated surgeries, and it is quickly becoming the norm for treating acute exacerbations of chronic and terminal conditions. Since intensive care beds have been increasingly available in many facilities, the criteria for admission have been lowered. Thus, the growing number of beds has influenced clinical decision making toward the use of intensive care whenever it may be helpful.

Concern about this growing use has led us to research on the types of patients receiving intensive care and the degree to which they are benefitting. Knaus et al. found that there were two types of patients who did not seem to derive much benefit from treatment in an intensive care unit. 3 Patients admitted for routine monitoring (20%), who were at such low risk that their ICU admissions could have been deferred, constituted one group. A second group included those admitted for cardiovascular and respiratory support, even though death was imminent.

It is unclear whether patients who are expected to die soon actually use large amounts of intensive care resources to little avail. Knaus et al. found that patients with written Do Not Resuscitate (DNR) orders used 13 percent of ICU resources before, and 3 percent after, the order was written. A somewhat different picture emerges from another study. Youngner found that ICU patients who were ultimately declared DNR were the highest consumers of resources, both before and after the orders were written.

Since the elderly constitute a large percentage of those treated in intensive care, questions have been raised about their utilization patterns and clinical decisions made regarding their care. Although elderly patients do not stay in intensive care longer than younger patients, they do require more interventions and have a lower survivai rate (for example, there is 44% mortality for those over 65 years old, as opposed to 21.8% for those aged 55-64). Elderly patients are generally admitted to intensive care for exacerbations of chronic conditions, rather than acute illness. The fact that charges for younger nonsurvivors in one study were higher than those for elderly nonsurvivors suggests that the most aggressive treatment may be reserved for younger patients. Decisions to limit use of intensive care may also be inferred from the finding that the 5.2 percent of ICU patients who entered from nursing homes did not differ greatly from the population over 65 in nursing homes. Given the chronically ill nature and high mortality of the nursing home population, one would expect nursing home transfers to account for a higher percentage of ICU admissions, if most of the seriously ill or dying patients in this group were admitted. It is likely that hospital and nursing home clinicians make decisions to not treat all patients aggressively.

The degree to which the high costs of intensive care produce positive outcomes is important in determining the justification for intensive care. Studies have demonstrated the effectiveness of intensive care for respiratory failure and other selected groups of critically ill patients. For example, Wagner found that study patients classified as being the most severely ill consumed large amounts of resources in intensive care units, but received treatments that could not have been given on the wards. The two-month mortality rate for these patients was 54 percent.

It is disconcerting, however, to discover that the costs of intensive care are often highest for those with the worst outcomes. Knaus found that the most severely ill patients constituted only 4 percent of the ICU admissions, but consumed 8 percent of the resources; most of them (92%) died within six months of hospitalization. Another study found that the most critically ill and costly patients had a oneyear death rate of 73 percent. When the same study was performed eight years carlier, this group had a similar death rate, suggesting that improved technology had not affected the outcome. Parno et al. found that hospital charges were highest for those patients who died in the hospital after spending time in the ICU. In fact, there seems to be a U-shaped relationship between intensive carc costs and the probability of death. Using a severity of illness measure on 613 consecutive admissions to the ICU, Scheffler et al. identified three groups of patients. Forty-five percent of the admissions used 19 percent of the total resources consumed, with the probability of death decreasing as resource consumption increased; their diagnoses were mainly acute, including ketoacidosis, cardiac arrest, and reversible shock. Another 46 percent of the patients were in a group in which the probability of death did not vary with resource consumption; this group consumed 57 percent of the resources. The other 9 percent of the patients consumed 24 percent of the resources, and the probability of death rose markedly with increased resource consumption.

Prognostic uncertainty also seems to contribute to high ICU costs. Detsky published a study which divided patients into survivors and nonsurvivors. The entire group of nonsurvivors cost more than survivors. Of the nonsurvivors, those with a good prognosis cost more than those with a clearly poor prognosis. These study findings suggest that clinicians are more likely to treat aggressively when a prognosis is uncertain, but there is some hope.

These studies reflect many of the current concerns about the high cost of intensive care relative to outcomes. Yet, the adequate assessment of the cost effectiveness of intensive care involves methodological problems. Studies that uncover the high costs of intensive care for particular groups of patients are based on charges for an episode of care—usually a hospital or ICU admission. There are several flaws in this approach. First, charges do not necessarily reflect resource consumption, especially in terms of nursing care. Patients receiving both intensive and routine care consume widely varying amounts of nursing time. In fact, ICU patients who receive routine monitoring may consume less personnel time than ward patients, a fact which is not reflected in the room charges. Routine monitoring patients cost less than their bed charges in intensive care, while sicker patients can cost much more than their charges. Traditional step-down methods of cost calculation do not take these differences in resource consumption into account. The flaw in this approach is that most studies use a hospital stay as the unit of analysis, rather than a patient's total consumption of health care in a given period. Because patients in intensive care typically have more costly stays, people tend to assume that they are the most costly group of patients in the health care system. Yet, studies that focus on the patient over time as the unit of analysis have found that the ICU patients cost less per year than chronic patients who are repeatedly admitted for routine care.14 Thus, while the per diem and per admission costs of intensive care patients are high and are rightly areas of concern, they should be viewed in the context of the total hospital costs, which may be more attributable to chronic, not critical, illness.

Despite the difficulties in assessing costs, there is still a question as to whether we devote more than the optimal amount of resources to intensive care. One useful approach to this issue might be a comparison of our intensive care expenditures with those in Great Britain and United States, where medical practice and science are similar. The per capita cost of British hospital care, after adjustment for salary differences, is less than one half of the cost in the United States. The supply of health care is controlled through a nationally fixed budget; primary care physicians control access to specialists in hospitals. There are one-fifth to one-tenth as many intensive care beds relative to the population in Great Britain as there are in U.S. hospitals. While British physicians generally report that they could use more intensive care beds, they believe this would pull resources from other needed programs. Despite these differences, life expectancy and general medical practice in the two countries are quite similar.

The preceding data suggest that the available technology and the related costs of intensive care are growing rapidly, and constitute a noteworthy portion of health care expenditures. Further, these expenditures may not always result in sufficient benefits. In order to understand the implications of this trend, one must be able to predict the future status of the population most at risk for receiving intensive care.

In the next few decades, rising life expectancy and a decline in mortality is expected to lead to higher morbidity, especially from the killer diseases. New advances in treatment will continue to lengthen the onset of the time between terminal phases of illness and death. Thus, the need for care of the critically and terminally ill is expected to increase in the short run, placing growing demand on intensive care units. In the long run, however, primary prevention of these killer diseases is expected to improve. Prevention will also lead to lowered mortality from killer diseases and higher prevalence rates for the chronic non-killer diseases—which will probably require more chronic, rather than critical, care. Thus, in the more distant future, chronic care needs are apt to compete more directly for critical care resources.

## ALLOCATION OF RESOURCES

Issues based on technological developments, high costs, growing numbers of both critically and chronically ill patients, and limits on societal resources devoted to health care will increasingly focus attention on both societal and institutional allocation of health care resources. Previously, however, there have been few restraints on the percentage of total health care allocated to intensive care, and little willingness to confront the reality of resource limits. In fact, the resources devoted to intensive care have increased, while preventive and primary care programs have been constrained. One reason for intensive care's immunity may be the fact that life-saving medical services are consistent with a societal view of human life as priceless. While individuals may "ignore health hazards and avoid prompt treatment of illness suggesting that they often value other outcomes more than health, not to do everything near the point of death is difficult to accept and still maintain a humanitarian self-image."

Another explanation for the discrepancy between the growth of intensive care and that of other types of programs is the distinction between identifiable and statistical lives. Preventive programs are usually designed and evaluated on the basis of epidemiological data and statistical evidence regarding the probabilities of illness under certain conditions. The thousands of children who will be impaired by inadequate prenatal diets and resulting low birthweight remain anonymous. On the other hand, the possibility of you or I or another critically ill person not receiving care that has even a remote chance of saving us brings us in direct symbolic contact with individuals and their mortality.

## Macroallocation

The importance we attach to the symbolic value of life-saving care is evidenced by our choices regarding resource macroallocation to health programs. Yankauer discusses this issue in relation to recent cutbacks in the women, infants, and children (WIC) program, a nutritional program for pregnant mothers and newborns. While other countries provide these types of basis services to all their citizens, we seem compelled to justify their extension with tax money in terms of direct results in other areas—such as reduced infant mortality. Yet, twice as much money has been spent on making the benefits of an endstage renal disease (ESRD) program universally available (that is, 1 billion on WIC as opposed to 2 billion on ESRD). Public and private insurance programs ensure the universal availability of coronary bypass operations. The existence of these services need not be justified by proving that they result in other benefits, such as greater employment or productivity. Our tendency not to question these infrequently used but very costly services is in direct opposition to our position on basic and less costly services.

The existence of these types of implicit macroallocation decisions is illustrated by a Hospital, where 30 percent of the women delivering infants have had no prenatal care. Yet, continued governmental cuts of prenatal programs are accompanied by the mandate that all efforts be made to save seriously ill newborns and provide neonatal intensive care.

The existence of a technological imperative in health care provides an additional explanation for the relatively unbridled growth of intensive care. A common viewpoint has been that if something can be done it should be done. Further, the technological treatment innovations provided in intensive care have not been subjected to the same controls as other types of treatments and programs. The widespread use of new drugs and food additives must be preceded by extremely rigorous experimental evidence of efficiency and safety. Social welfare programs, such as day care and employment training, are severely cut if cost-effective results cannot be demonstrated. The diffusion of medical technological innovations, on the other hand, is only subject to indirect control, primarily through the lack of immediate reimbursement for procedures which are considered experimental. Initial reimbursement, however, is not based on uniform demands for proof of efficacy or benefit.

Public resistance to direct confrontation of the possibility of limited resources for life-saving treatment is reflected in opinion polls that oppose medical care rationing, even for those with little hope of recovery; 61 percent were opposed in one survey. Yet, restrictive public policy suggests an unwillingness to completely assume the costs for those who are medically indigent. The difficulty in reconciling these inconsistent attitudes may partially account for the failure to openly consider the problems of resource allocation to critical care.

The experience with the end-stage renal disease program illustrates society's difficulty in making tough choices with regard to life-saving treatments. The government reacted to limited supplies of dialysis by making complete coverage for this disease a universal entitlement. While the enormous cost of this experience (with annual growth rate of 37% since inception) with an early life-saving technology suggests that this will not occur again, it does demonstrate how far our society will go to avoid the issue.

Despite the lack of direct efforts to control the development and growth of intensive care, there are several mechanisms that have the potential to affect its supply.

Certificate of need programs have attempted to control health care costs by restricting excessive or duplicative services. Although CON was a prerequisite for large capital expenditures in all states but Louisiana by 1980, it is difficult to detect any CON-related limitations on intensive care. In fact CON programs have apparently decreased the number of beds while increasing hospital assets per bed. Thus, there seem to have been general per them increases in costs and intensity of care. Only a few instances can be cited in which CON programs have controlled the growth of intensive care beds or other technology; such instances seem to result from the combination of a CON program and state rate-setting activities.

Since the need for intensive care is directly proportional to technological development, controlling the growth of technology can indirectly slow the growth of intensive care. Technological development can be reduced by limiting research funds, and there is some evidence that this is occurring at the govt. level. To the extent that intensive technologies are profitable; however, the private sector can be expected to invest in research and development efforts. Recent work on the artificial heart illustrates this type of private investment. Consideration is also being given to the use of a more thorough government review process as a means of controlling technology. Both new and existing technological innovations and procedures may be subjected to an effectiveness assessment prior to their adoption and reimbursement in the future.

Recent changes in health care financing are influencing hospitals' incentives for supplying intensive care. Prospective payment based on diagnostic-related groups (DRGS) currently includes no differential for ICU care. Yet, the cost of care in an intensive care unit may well exceed the payment levels for medical DRGs that most commonly occur in intensive care. Since patients receiving intensive care will produce financial losses for the hospital, the current payment system is likely to influence the supply of intensive care beds. Intensive care has flourished under a system in which the costs were more nearly reimbursable; in fact, cross-subsidization often resulted in payments that exceeded costs—for example, ancillary services. As funding continues to move in the direction of prospective payment, rather than cost reimbursement, hospital officials may decide that limiting the quantity of intensive care beds is preferable to attracting large numbers of critically ill patients and incurring financial loss.

The budgetary process in Great Britain effectively limits the availability of intensive care and other life-saving technologies—a practice that does not currently occur in the United States. This results in some clear patterns of resource allocation. There are more restrictions on care for the elderly than there are for the young. Life-saving treatments have been curtailed less than those that improve quality of life—that is, elective admissions to hospitals are delayed. Treatments involving expensive equipment or new technology are also restricted. These limits are subtly manifested in physician behavior and practice patterns. Physicians, for example, do not recommend dialysis for older patients or those with other serious complications. Patients accept these recommendations with little question because they are consistent with standard medical practice. Although physicians justify decisions not to institute or to discontinue aggressive treatments as medically appropriate, they also seem cognizant of supply restrictions. Thus, the standards of medical practice have been adjusted to conform to the constraints imposed by limited resources.

The rising level of debate and discussion suggests increasing recognition of the fact that health care resources are not unlimited; doing more of one thing may mean having to do less of something else. Yet, difficult ethical and political concerns are involved in addressing these dilemmas of macroallocation. Many new questions of equity, fairness, and feasibility arise. Should a technology be available to all with equal need, or, are there some basic types of services that should be guaranteed for all, beyond which the individual would assume responsibility. Gutmann argued that "a principle of equal access to health care demands that every person who shares the same type and degree of health need must be given an equally effective chance of receiving appropriate treatment of equal quality so long as that treatment is available to anyone." This suggests that while society is not obligated to provide any particular intensity of care, all persons with similar needs must have an equally effective chance of receiving any available high technology services, such as heart transplants. Such a principle places limits upon freedom of purchase, especially for the wealthiest members of our society.

Currently available methods of controlling expenditures on intensive care also pose ethical problems. Limitations which only apply to new technology and are enforced by payment restrictions could result in an inequity—in other words, there would be no restrictions on people needing older technologies, while those who could possibly benefit from new technologies would face limitations. For example, most people with kidney disease could be saved, but those with liver disease could not.

Using prospective payment to control intensity of care also poses dilemmas. Because the current method provides incentives for hospitals to treat the healthiest patients within each DRG, those who require costly treatments, such as intensive care, may be avoided. While holding down costs, this method would create a system in which those with the greatest need might actually receive the least care. This undesirable effect could be diminished by adjusting prospective payment to reflect severity of illness differences within DRGS. If patients with more serious illnesses, who are presumably in greater need of intensive care, are paid accordingly, they might take priority for ICU admission over those who are less ill.

While the thought of limiting the growth of intensive care raises immediate concerns about equity and restriction of liberty, the failure to limit intensive care in the face of scarce health care resources also produces ethical dilemmas.

The fact that intensive care has been made widely available with little regard to age or health status suggests that our society has opted for extending life whenever possible. To the degree that this has restricted our ability to fund other types of programs, we may have reduced the possibility of maximizing the length and quality of life for all, while extending it for a few who become critically ill. Thus, the issue may really involve allocation for either preventive medicine or life-prolonging care. From one perspective, prevention may be a more effective means of raising the general level of health and quality of life. But it could lead to the neglect of needy persons who could directly benefit from the resources of intensive care. Resolving this issue requires weighing the goal of maximum costefficiency against the costly needs of a relatively small number of individuals.

## Microallocation

It seems inevitable that the resources available for health care will be restricted. Within these limitations, it also seems likely that the supply of expensive technologies, such as intensive care, will be constrained. These facts raise the problem of how the available intensive care resources should be distributed. How much should go to which technologies and which patients. How will this rationing be implemented, and how will hospitals, physicians, and patients react.

Methods of allocating any scarce resource, such as intensive care, typically reflect one or more principles of distribution. The principles may be implicit or explicit; they may or may not be defensible from an ethical point of view or be practical to implement. Commonly cited justifications for distributing scarce societal resources to certain individuals include:

- The person's merit or past contributions;
- Tvercoming past wrongs done to the person (e.g., compensatory programs);
- Severity of need;

- The amount of effort or other resources the person can exchange for services;
- An effort to distribute the resource equitably;
- An effort to produce the greatest good for society.

There is already some implicit rationing with regard to intensive care. Resource allocation at several levels determines whether a patient with a life-threatening condition receives intensive care. First, does the patient reach a hospital that offers intensive care. The geographic distribution of intensive care units and the patient's medical insurance status may determine the answer to this question. For example, there are currently fewer intensive care beds in rural areas, public hospitals, and hospitals that serve the poor. Further, if the patient is either institutionalized or being cared for in the home, the providers' decisions about patient transfer may actually determine whether intensive care is received. Second, is the hospitalized patient admitted to an intensive care unit. The answer will be partially based on whether the patient's medical condition is judged serious enough to require intensive care and the possibility of benefit from intensive care. It will further be affected by the availability of an intensive care bed; if no bed is available, the decision will depend on whether this patient's need or potential to benefit is greater or lesser than those of other patients. It could also be affected by nonmedical considerations, such as patient and family preferences, judgments about the patient's social value, or the patient's financial situation.

Finally, what treatments are provided to the patient in the ICU. Although treatment decisions typically depend upon the patient's present medical condition, they are also influenced by prognosis, patient and family wishes, and staff reactions to caring for the patient. Treatment limitations may manifest themselves in the form of an explicit order, such as "do not resuscitate," or in a series of choices to not do everything possible.

At every point in this rationing process, several questions can be raised. First, are the decisions based on accurate facts and adequate analysis of the facts. Most problematic in this regard are attempts to estimate prognoses and predict the benefits to be gained from intensive care in general, as well as specific treatments. This aspect of decision making may be facilitated by protocols and indices which predict severity of illness, occurrence of complications, probability of mortality, and future functioning. Technological assessments and studies of treatment effectiveness will contribute to clinicians' ability to make these judgments accurately.

Second, are the decisions ethical. The ethical nature of these decisions is often viewed from the perspectives of the individual patient and clinician. When examined in this manner, the ethical concerns focus on protecting patient autonomy, fulfilling the clinician's obligation to do all that is best for the patient, and the clinician's duty to inform the patient about treatment options and their effects. However, because these decisions involve scarce resources, what is done for one patient will affect what can be done for other patients. Thus, the decisions must be examined simultaneously from the perspectives of patient groups and society as a whole. When this point of view is adopted, the major ethical consideration involves social justice, which asks whether patterns of treatment decisions are consistent with values such as fairness, equity, liberty, and maximum benefits for all.

Third, how can these decisions be made practically. What processes of clinical and patient decision making will facilitate both accurate factual analysis and ethical behaviors or outcomes.

Although rationing guidelines have seldom been made explicit, several implicit forms of health care rationing do exist. Using a method based on economics, a limited resource is given only to those who can pay. Thus, government financing, third party payor decisions, and the societal distribution of wealth actually determine who receives the service. Rationing based on economics occurs in intensive care when patients with little or no insurance are denied hospital admission, not scheduled for elective procedures, or die outside the hospital from conditions for which individuals with better insurance coverage would have been under medical supervision. The theory that the market is the most efficient allocator of resources has many supporters; it is often argued that this theory is not applicable to health care because limited knowledge or finances prevent many people from satisfying their desires through the marketplace.

A second method of implicit rationing is manifested in practical and administrative decisions. For example, a person will not be moved from an intensive care bed because another patient is waiting (that is, first-come-first-served). Another illustration involves the provision of slightly less nursing time for each patient when the supply of nursing resources is short (that is, equal rationing).

A third rationing mechanism is based on nonmedical patient characteristics, some of which may reflect "social value." The limited supply of intensive care in rural areas serves to limit its availability to rural residents. There are also examples of rationing on the basis of race. The use of socioeconomic status as an implicit criterion for rationing medical care is exemplified by an examination of transfers from private to public hospitals. Ten percent of those transferred were found to be seriously jeopardized by the move; most of those transferred were young, uninsured, and minority patients.

Rationing based on health status or need has seldom been made explicit, but is reflected in norms and practice patterns within institutions. Needs assessment can affect resource provision in two directions. Those with the most severe illnesses may be given the most resources because their needs are greatest; alternatively, they may be given fewer resources, because the benefit to them and society is judged to be minimal. For example, patients with DNR orders or terminally ill patients may receive fewer life-saving treatments or be denied admission to intensive care units. While not explicitly documented, decisions to forego specific life-sustaining treatment interventions (for example, dialysis, transfusions, antibiotics, hyperalimentation, and others) are sometimes made for patients whose condition is deemed hopeless.

In Great Britain, where resource limits have been acknowledged for some time, physicians implement rationing of care on the basis of health status. Certain expensive treatments are just not recommended for certain patients; for example, renal dialysis is considered inadvisable for older patients. The system makes denial of care seem routine and even optimal.

Effective rationing on the basis of health status requires precise predictions of the benefits of particular treatments for particular patients. Recent investigations have focused on the degree to which various patients can be expected to benefit from intensive care. Attempts have been made to assess the risk of complications for patients who are often admitted to ICUs for monitoring. For example, a protocol developed to aid in acute chest pain diagnosis has substantially increased the efficiency of ICU admissions. The protocol reduced the number of false positive ICU admissions, while increasing the true negatives and maintaining the true positive rate. The experience at Massachusetts General Hospital suggests the potential savings that may result from reduced monitoring admissions. When the number of intensive care beds was temporarily reduced, low-risk patients were not admitted to the ICU—with no negative results.

Identifying patients who have an extremely poor chance of hospital survival regardless of care intensity is another means of resource rationing based on health status. Single factors or diagnostic categories have not been successful in identifying subgroups of patients with a high probability of death. However, APACHE, a multiattributable measure of severity of illness, has proven to be a good predictor of ICU mortality and resource consumption within selected diagnostic categories. A much more controversial approach to rationing care would involve the assessment of future quality of life if the patient survives the ICU stay.

Another means of resource rationing is to limit treatment for patients already in the ICU. Little is known about how clinicians decide to institute or cease specific treatments. For example, some studies suggest that resource expenditures may be reduced when patients are declared DNR, while others find no such limitation. With the exception of cardiopulmonary resuscitation, where factors predicting nonsurvival have been identified, few guidelines are available for specific procedures.

Terminal illness, an indicator of health status, makes patients ineligible for ICU admission in a few places, but this is not the norm. While patients have a right to refuse life-sustaining treatment, circumstances or the patient's own condition often preclude the effective exercise of this right. In the absence of a clear and cogent request not to do so, physicians often feel obligated to "do everything." Critics ask whether these cases result in an unreasonable amount of resource expenditures.1,16 Some hospitals have used a classification of terminally ill patients to indicate the degree of treatment to be instituted when life is threatened. Levels range from those patients who are eligible for cardiopulmonary resuscitation and all other interventions to those who should receive only general nursing, hydration, nutrition, and comfort measures. While the importance of patient and family involvement in decision making is stressed, the influence of the options presented by the physician is recognized.

Implicit or explicit rationing of intensive care entails clinical, ethical, and legal dilemmas. Clinicians often seem reluctant to use statistical predictors of health status to determine care, even if past experience predicts 100 percent mortality. The rationale is that while survival may be unprecedented, it may not be impossible. Studies also suggest that human decision makers are limited in their abilities to simultaneously process multiple criteria and their related probabilities. Further, even when denial or termination of care is clinically, ethically, and legally justifiable, the emotional reactions of caregivers and family affect clinical decisions.

The individual clinician who must make rationing decisions is faced with a psychological and ethical struggle. The clinician's relationship with the patient involves ethical obligations; yet these duties to the individual patient invariably conflict with societal considerations. Because it results from resource scarcity, the concept of rationing must use society, as opposed to the individual, as the unit of analysis. Thus, guidelines for allocation of intensive care resources must be developed when one is not confronting an individual patient in need. Explicit criteria are essential to the promotion of practice patterns that are consistent with an ethical distribution of scarce resources.

The predominant ethical question applicable to general criteria for rationing intensive care, as opposed to bedside decision making about individual patients, is the degree to which the use of the criteria result in a just distribution of resources. A review of alternative conceptualizations of distributive justice is beyond the scope of this book. However, two somewhat contrasting viewpoints are frequently offered in discussions of the ethical aspects of rationing. One focuses on a utilitarian or cost-benefit consideration, and the other focuses on equity.

From a utilitarian perspective, methods of rationing intensive care would be considered just if they resulted in the greatest total amount of benefit to all—that is, the greatest good for the greatest number. In other words, treatment should be given to those critically ill individuals most likely to exhibit positive results—for example, survival, improved functioning, reduced morbidity, maximum life satisfaction, productivity, or any other outcomes judged to be desirable by both the individuals involved and society as a whole. At the same time, caring for these individuals should not interfere with the provision of care that produces more total benefits to society. Triage, as practiced in battlefield medicine, is an example of a rationing procedure that seems consistent with a utilitarian view. Patients who are critically injured but also most likely to recover following treatment are given priority over those whose injuries are less immediately dangerous or those with poor prognoses. Although the utilitarian conception of justice has received considerable attention and explication, its use in judging criteria for rationing intensive care is problematic. Critics of utilitarianism, including John Rawls, note that the concept is fraught with both practical and moral problems. The practical problem entails the quantification and aggregation of the total benefits that would accrue from the distribution of a resource in a certain way. The total benefits cannot be calculated by considering the gross numbers of people helped; consideration must also be given to what else could have been done with the resources. It is difficult to compare the benefits accruing to ten people who each receive 50 days of ICU care with those of 100 people who receive five days each. It is also difficult to judge how much a day of extended life for a patient may affect the total benefits to family and society. Simply stated, the greatest good for the greatest number principle lacks an operational method for determining the relative benefits of resources for different groups of people.

There are also moral problems within the utilitarian view. It has been argued that defining justice as that which produces the greatest good for the greatest number enables societal tolerance of the exploitation or suffering of a small minority—even, for example, an institution as abhorrent as slavery. The application of this principle to intensive care might dictate the nontreatment of a few very costly critically ill patients for whom death was imminent, even if the patients strongly desired a few more days of life. Such practice conflicts with the value placed on patient autonomy and rights. The utilitarian principle is typically applied within the context of other competing or higher order principles. In Mill's original work on utilitarianism, the accompanying principle was the concept of "maximum liberty for all." In current discussions of intensive care, the goals of maximizing patient autonomy and preserving the physician's duty to act in ways that benefit the patient are essential. Rationing criteria that reflect utilitarian considerations would, therefore, need to be combined with methods for eliciting the patient's own judgments of benefits and affirming the duties of health care providers.

The egalitarian perspective for judging rationing mechanisms places priority on the value of equity—specifically, to what extent does the method of distributing resources treat individuals equitably. , Equitable treatment should not be confused with equal treatment. Equal treatment, such as that which is characteristic of a first-come-first-served or lottery approach, may also be just if peoples' needs and abilities to claim resources are equal. However, equal treatment will seldom be equitable with respect to intensive care because people differ markedly in their need for, and access to, intensive care. The egalitarian principle put forward by Rawls argues that people should generally be treated equally. Unequal treatment is justified if it benefits the most needy or disadvantaged. In the case of intensive care, this suggests that people whose needs are similar be treated equally; when resources are scarce, those with the greatest needs are to be benefitted. Approaches to rationing which are consistent with a cost-benefit perspective but restrict access to a particular life-saving technology, such as the artificial heart, may be questioned on the basis of an equity principle (that is, all those with equal need do not receive hearts).

Need assessment constitutes the major practical difficulty in judging rationing mechanisms according to their contribution to equity. While progress has been made in measuring deviation from normal physiological status, there are currently no methods for assessing the patient's subjective experience of being critically ill. The patient's degree of suffering, discomfort, distress, and anxiety would certainly be an essential component of need under a system that allows unequal treatment when it benefits the most disadvantaged.

Several aspects of the egalitarian perspective present ethical difficulties. Those who have the greatest need are likely to be in an extremely deteriorated condition. Despite their consumption of vast amounts of resources, many of these individuals would die, leaving other less severely ill individuals without access to critical care. Further, this principle might impose inordinate demands upon all health care resources, thus restricting the supply of more basic types of primary and preventive care.

Proponents of a libertarian view are likely to criticize both egalitarian and utilitarian allocation schemes for intensive care. Allocation of valued resources on the basis of need or potential benefit would interfere with the unrestricted exchange of the marketplace, in which individuals freely exchange their holdings. Libertarians would argue that those individuals who place the greatest value on intensity of care in the event of their own critical illnesses could freely choose to insure themselves for such eventualities, thereby guaranteeing unlimited access. It would be argued that these individual choices should not be restricted by any rationing mechanisms.

While ethical and practical dilemmas make rationing intensive care difficult to contemplate, fear of malpractice litigation has probably been a more direct determinant of its unrestricted use. The tendency to believe that technology can solve most problems, and to respond to failure by seeking to pinpoint blame or liability, has been cited as a factor that would make open rationing extremely risky. The perceived threat of a lawsuit is often cited as a reason for patients being admitted to ICUs for monitoring. However, clearer monitoring and ICU admission criteria would be likely to set new standards of medical practice; this would lower concern about malpractice, which is typically defined as deviation from the norm. It is instructive to note that little malpractice litigation has resulted from the prevalent rationing in Great Britain. One explanation for this phenomenon is the fact that British attorneys require payment for handling these cases regardless of the outcome; contingency fees are not allowed. Also, malpractice suits are typically based on the argument that the patient received care that deviated from standard medical practice. In Great Britain, where ICU care is not the standard for many conditions, failure to provide it is not judged as deviant. Therefore, this argument is not the basis for successful litigation.

## CONCLUSIONS

It seems clear that unrestricted consumption of health care resources in critical illness conflicts with other health and welfare needs within society. Changes in payment mechanisms for hospital care and new developments in technology assessment and control suggest that we will soon experience limits on the availability of intensive care. This supply restriction can be attributed to the rising demands created by the population's aging and the increased life span of the chronically and terminally ill. These trends will inevitably lead to recognition of the need to ration intensive care.

In rationing intensive care, it will be necessary to create a balance between explicit criteria that guard against discrimination and promote distributive justice, and implicit judgments that allow some consideration of unique or subjective factors. Reducing ICU admissions of patients who need only routine monitoring and are at low risk for complications seems to be a promising area for rationing criteria which are consistent with both egalitarian and utilitarian views of justice. Limiting care for patients who have little potential for survival or quality of life is another potential area for saving substantial resources.

Although restricting the development of new but expensive life-saving technologies also promises to reduce expenditures, this will be more controversial from an ethical point of view.

Decision makers in ICUs would be better able to deal with the problem of rationing if there were less uncertainty regarding prognosis and expected benefits of care. Studies of the natural history of intensive care illnesses, as well as studies that pinpoint clinical predictors for patients at high risk of complications, would help in this regard.

The organizational structure of ICUs will also affect the ability to allocate resources fairly. The use of something other than a first-comefirst-served or random approach requires a comparative view of needs, benefits, and demands across a population. Equitable rationing (that is, allocation) would require ICU directors who could consider all patients in decision making, rather than just their own.

Public policy and the health benefits policies of employers and insurers will provide a context in which medical center rationing will take place. Policy changes, such as the recent use of DRGs for prospective payment, are often implemented with little consideration of their potential effect on the allocation of intensive care. Yet, these effects may be serious, and need to be analyzed in terms of their distributional consequences.

Any mechanisms for allocating intensive care will work only insofar as they have widespread support. Thus, rationing criteria cannot produce situations that seem outrageous, upsetting, or unfair to clinicians, patients, or the public at large. The experience in Britain is an example of an evolved consensus, in which the practice patterns developed in response to limits are generally accepted; the extraordinary is neither desired nor considered reasonable by most people. Most people would have difficulty accepting the limited availability of intensive care. However, despite this lack of acceptance, the process of managing scarce intensive care resources seems to be underway, and will require research, scholarly analysis, and public debate. Clinicians, researchers, philosophers, social scientists, politicians, and consumers will all be involved in the evolving system of intensive care allocation.

# Chapter 6

# Practical Proceduress

## GENERAL INFORMATION

Patients in intensive care often require large numbers of practical procedures. The information in this chapter is intended only as a guide. The advice is generalized; you should always read the instructions provided with the equipment that you use, and follow your local hospital guidelines.

### Consent

Formal consent/assent may be appropriate for some procedures, such as tracheostomy, while consent/assent may be implied for minor or life-saving procedures. In any event, always explain to patients, even if apparently 'unconscious', what you intend to do and keep relatives informed.

### Local Anaesthetic

Paralysed and sedated patients in ICU may still feel pain from invasive procedures. Use local anaesthetic for all painful procedures.

### Universal infection control precautions

Contamination with blood imposes significant risk to staff from blood-borne infection, particularly hepatitis and HIV infection. Universal precautions should be adopted for all invasive procedures. These are intended to prevent the spread of infection, to protect you, your patients and colleagues. It is not always possible to know who has an infection; universal infection control precautions apply to everybody, all of the time:

- Wash your hands thoroughly.
- Cuts or grazes on the hands or forearms should be covered with a waterproof dressing while at work. Seek medical advice about any septic or weeping areas.
- Single-use gloves should be worn for direct contact with blood or body fluid, broken skin or mucous membranes. Face protection and plastic aprons should be worn if there is a risk of blood or body fluid splashing the face or clothing.
- Place all sharps directly into a sharps bin; do not manually resheath or break needles. Do not overfill sharps bins, and ensure that the bin is securely fastened before disposal.

If you do accidentally cut, scrape or puncture your skin, follow the 'accidental inoculation procedure', i.e.

- Encourage bleeding, wash with warm soapy water, dry and cover with a waterproof dressing.
- Report the incident to the senior person in charge and ensure a report is completed.
- Seek advice from the occupational health department or from A and E.

Clinical waste should be discarded into colour-coded bags for incineration. Blood or body fluid spills should be disinfected immediately; follow instructions.

Always follow guidelines and safety information that apply to your department. If you need further information, talk in the first place to a senior member of staff. Where necessary, further advice can be obtained from specialists in microbiology, infection control, occupational health, health & safety, etc.

### Aseptic Technique

ICU patients are generally severely debilitated and at increased risk of infection; therefore, when performing procedures, no matter how minor, good infection control procedures are important. For all invasive procedures strict aseptic technique is required:

- Collect all necessary equipment before starting.
- Ensure assistance is available to open packs, etc.
- Wash hands with disinfectant (generally chlorhexidine or iodine).
- Dry hands on towel provided in gown pack.
- Put on gown.
- Put on gloves using closed technique.
- Prepare the equipment on the trolley.
- Prepare the patient by washing with spirit or iodine.
- Place sterile towels around the proposed site to make a sterile field.
- Remember to keep hands up to avoid contamination.

## ARTERIAL CANNULATION

Arterial cannulation is one of the most commonly performed procedures in the ICU. There is, however, an associated risk of morbidity and the indication for arterial cannulation in the individual patient should be considered carefully.

### Indications

Haemodynamic monitoring:

- Particularly in situations where noninvasive measurements are inadequate, e.g. where changes in arterial blood pressure are likely to be sudden or profound, at extremes of blood pressure and in the presence of arrhythmias.
- Repeated blood sampling. Especially for repeated arterial blood gas sampling. The complications associated with arterial cannulation are outweighed by the morbidity and inconvenience of repeated arterial puncture.

### Contraindications

These are relative. Exercise caution in arteriopaths and do not recannulate an artery where previous vascular compromise has occurred. Where possible avoid areas of local sepsis and trauma, limbs with dialysis fistulae and end arteries such as the brachial artery.

### Procedure

Decide which artery to cannulate. The radial artery of the nondominant hand is usually preferred in the first instance. Alternatives include the ulnar, dorsalis pedis and posterior tibial arteries. It is pointless, however, to persist with attempts at peripheral arterial cannulation in patients who are hypotensive and 'shut down'. The femoral and brachial arteries are useful during resuscitation of profoundly shocked patients.

Arterial cannulation often results in blood spillage. Universal precautions should be used.

Clean the puncture site and establish a sterile field.

Gently palpate the artery and inject local anaesthetic to raise a small intradermal bleb at the puncture site 1 cm distal to the proposed cannulation site.

A Seldinger technique or a direct cannulation technique may be used.

### *Seldinger technique*

Advance needle through the puncture site towards the artery at a shallow angle. As the vessel is punctured, a flashback of arterial blood is seen in the hub. Pass the guide wire through the needle into the artery. Withdraw the needle and pass the cannula over the guide wire. The guide wire is then discarded.

### *Direct cannulation*

Either: advance the cannula and needle through the puncture site towards the artery at a shallow angle. As the vessel is punctured a flashback of arterial blood is seen in the hub. Holding the needle still, advance the cannula over the needle into the artery. This should be a single smooth movement without resistance.

Or: advance the cannula at a steeper angle and, after observing the flashback, continue through the artery to transfix it. Withdraw the needle slightly from the cannula and then pull the cannula back gently until the tip is in the artery and flashback is again observed.

Advance the cannula into the artery.

Attach extension tubing and three-way tap.

Aspirate blood from the line to confirm placement and to remove any air bubbles, then flush line with heparinized saline.

Secure in place and cover with occlusive dressing. (If using stitches, do not place stitches too deeply. It is possible inadvertently to damage peripheral arteries.) Attach the arterial catheter to a pressure transducer and flushing device.

## Sampling from Arterial Lines

Clean sample port with alcohol swab and attach syringe.

Aspirate 1–2 ml blood into the syringe and then discard this syringe.

Aspirate sample into fresh syringe or vacuum container.

Samples for blood gases should be drawn into preheparinized syringes to prevent damage to the blood gas analyser. Any air in the syringe should be expelled. If not analysed immediately in the ICU, the syringe should be capped and placed on ice.

Flush the line with heparinized saline and place a clean cap on the sampling port.

## Complications

Complications of arterial cannulation are discussed. Vascular compromise may occur at any stage. Inadvertent injection of drugs into an arterial catheter is an important avoidable cause of morbidity and all cannulae and lines should be clearly labelled. Risk of infection increases with time. Any manifestly infected catheter should be removed. After removal press firmly for at least 5 minutes. Occasionally persistent bleeding may require a suture (5/0 nylon) to close the skin wound and then further pressure.

A transducer converts one type of energy (e.g. arterial pressure) into another (e.g. electrical impulse). There are a number of different types of transducer available but the principle is similar for all:

- The patient's arterial catheter is connected to the transducer by a continuous column of heparinized saline. A pressurized flushing device maintains a small forward flow (approx. 2–3 ml/h) to keep the cannula patent.
- Pressure changes in the vessel are transmitted via the saline to a diaphragm.

## PRESSURE TRANSDUCERS

A transducer converts one type of energy (e.g. arterial pressure) into another (e.g. electrical impulse). There are a number of different types of transducer available but the principle is similar for all:

- The patient's arterial catheter is connected to the transducer by a continuous column of heparinized saline. A pressurized flushing device maintains a small forward flow (approx. 2–3 ml/h) to keep the cannula patent.

- Pressure changes in the vessel are transmitted via the saline to a diaphragm. As this diaphragm moves in response to the pressure changes, its electrical conductivity changes. This results in fluctuations in electrical signal from the diaphragm, which is interpreted by a monitor and displayed as an arterial waveform and blood pressure values. Systolic, diastolic and mean pressures are usually displayed.

### Using Transducers

In order for the arterial waveform and blood pressure recording to be accurate, the transducer must be used appropriately. Therefore:

- There must be no air bubble in the connection tubing or transducer chamber. This will damp the trace and produce lower blood pressure values. Flush well before connecting the transducer to the patient.

- The transducer should be maintained at the level of the left atrium and appropriately zeroed. (If raised above this level the recorded pressure will be too low, and vice versa.)

### Zeroing Transducers

To zero a transducer turn the three-way tap so the transducer is open to air and the patient connection is switched off. The transducer is now connected to atmospheric or zero gauge pressure.

Zero the monitoring system according to the manufacturer's instructions. (There is usually a single button to press.)

When zeroing is complete, turn the three-way tap back to reconnect the patient to the transducer. Check that the trace and values obtained are as expected.

## COMMON PROBLEMS: INVASIVE PRESSURE MONITORING

### Invasive and Non-Invasive Pressures Disagree

If the blood pressure displayed by the invasive arterial monitoring differs from that obtained by non-invasive methods this is usually the result of either damping or resonance in the invasive monitoring. In most cases the mean arterial pressures are usually in close agreement.

Check the arterial line is correctly sited and flush the lumen with heparinized saline.

Check that there are no air bubbles in the connecting tubing or transducer chamber.

Check zero on invasive monitoring.

Check that the transducer is at the level of the left atrium. In some cases, peripheral vasospasm may be a cause of this error. If in doubt, resite the arterial line, or use the non-invasive measurements of blood pressure. In this case, the line can still be retained for arterial blood gas sampling.

### Indications

Central venous access is almost universal in intensive care patients. Indications include:

- Monitoring of CVP
- Drug administration
- Total parenteral nutrition
- Fluid resuscitation
- Insertion of temporary pacing wires
- Insertion of pulmonary artery catheters Dialysis
- Lack of peripheral venous access.

**Contraindications**

These are relative but include inability to identify landmarks, limited sites for access, previous difficulties or complications, severe coagulopathy, thrombocytopenia and local sepsis. In addition, if an awake patient is unable to lie flat, central venous cannulation may be impractical.

**Ultrasound Guidance for Vascular Access**

It is now increasingly recommended that ultrasound should be used to guide all central venous access. Ultrasound allows:

- Direct visualization of the vessels (artery and vein) and their associated structures
- Identification of thrombosis, valve or anatomical abnormalities
- Identification of best target vessel
- First-pass cannulation in the midline of a vessel directly avoiding other vital structures
- Visualization of guide wire and cannulae entering vein
- Reduction of puncture-related complications.

Arteries can be distinguished from veins by their round cross-section, non-compressibility and their pulsatility. Veins, by contrast, show respiratory fluctuation and are easily compressible. In order to maintain sterility during vessel puncture the ultrasound probe can be placed in a sterile plastic sheath. (Sterile ultrasound gel is required both inside and outside the sheath.) The use of ultrasound requires practice. You should seek instruction before attempting to use it on a patient. You should also be familiar with the landmark approaches to the central veins described below.

**Internal Jugular Vein**

Internal jugular vein cannulation is associated with a lower incidence of complications and higher incidence of correct line placement than other approaches. It is especially appropriate for patients with coagulopathy or those patients with lung disease in whom pneumothorax may be disastrous. It may be best avoided in those patients with carotid artery disease or those with raised intracranial pressure because of the risks of carotid puncture and of impaired cerebral venous drainage. Internal jugular cannulation is associated with a higher incidence of catheter infection than subclavian cannulation but both have a much lower infection rate than the femoral approach.

The internal jugular vein runs from the jugular foramen at the base of the skull (immediately behind the ear) to its termination behind the posterior border of the sternoclavicular joint where it combines with the subclavian vein to become the brachiocephalic vein. Throughout its length it lies lateral, first to the internal and then common carotid arteries, within the carotid sheath, behind the sternomastoid muscle.

Many approaches to the internal jugular vein have been described. Ultrasound will demonstrate the close association of the vein and carotid artery. Choose a site for puncture where the vein does not lie directly over the artery. A typical approach is from the apex of the triangle formed by the two heads of the sternomastoid:

- Slightly extend the neck.
- Turn the head slightly to the opposite side.
- Palpate the carotid artery at the level of the cricoid cartilage.
- Look for the internal jugular vein pulsation. If compressed, the internal jugular can usually be seen to empty and refill.
- To locate the vein, introduce needle from the apex of the triangle at an angle of 30° and aim towards the ipsilateral nipple.

Often when attempting to puncture the vein it collapses under the pressure of the needle and puncture is not recognized. The vessel may then be located by aspirating as the needle is slowly withdrawn. Blood will be aspirated as the needle tip passes back into the vein, which refills once the pressure has been removed.

## External Jugular Vein

The external jugular vein lies superficially in the neck, running down from the region of the angle of the jaw, across the sternomastoid before passing deep to drain into the subclavian vein. It can be used to provide central venous access, particularly in emergency situations when a simple large-bore cannula can be used for the administration of drugs and resuscitation fluids. Longer central venous catheters can be sited via the external jugular but the angle of entry to the subclavian vein often leads to inability to pass guide wires centrally and results in a high failure rate.

## Subclavian Vein

Subclavian vein cannulation is associated with a higher incidence of complications, particularly pneumothorax, and a higher incidence of incorrect line placement than internal jugular cannulation. It is, however, more comfortable for the patient long-term and the site can more easily be kept clean.

The subclavian vein is a continuation of the axillary vein. It runs from the apex of the axilla behind the posterior border of the clavicle and across the first rib to join the internal jugular vein, forming the brachiocephalic vein behind the sternoclavicular joint.

Position the patient supine (some people advocate placing a sandbag between the patient's shoulder blades, which allows the shoulders to drop back out of the way).

Identify the junction of medial third and outer two-thirds of the clavicle.

Introduce the needle just beneath the clavicle at this point, and aim towards the clavicle until contact with bone is made.

To locate the vein, redirect the needle closely behind the clavicle and towards the suprasternal notch.

Ultrasound can be used to guide puncture of the vein using a more lateral approach. The axillary vein can be identified in the apex of the axilla at a depth of 3–4 cm in the average patient. Longer catheters (20 cm left and 25 cm right) are required by this approach.

**Femoral Vein**

The femoral vein lies medial to the femoral artery immediately beneath the inguinal ligament. It is particularly useful for obtaining central access in small children and in patients with severe coagulopathy.

Palpate the femoral artery.

To locate the vein, introduce the needle 1 cm medial to the femoral artery close to the inguinal ligament. It is a common mistake to go too low where the superficial femoral artery overlies the vein.

Ultrasound can be used to identify the vessels and ensure that the vein is punctured near the inguinal ligament where the artery and vein lie side by side.

**Procedure**

Central venous catheterization is almost universally achieved using a catheter over a guide wire (Seldinger) technique. This is associated with a lower incidence of incorrect line placement and complications than cannula over needle techniques.

For internal jugular, external jugular and subclavian veins position the patient supine with 10–20° head down tilt. This distends the vein to aid location and helps prevent air embolism.

Monitor ECG in case of dysrhythmias (a defibrillator should be immediately available).

Universal precautions.

Use aseptic technique, sterile gown and gloves.

Prepare sterile field.

Prepare all equipment.

Check wire passes through the needle freely. Attach three-way taps to all open ports of the cannula. Flush the lumens with heparinized saline.

Inject local anaesthetic to the entry site. Do not forget to anaesthetize suture sites as well.

Identify the target vessel by ultrasound and/or landmark technique.

Using a 10-ml syringe (partially filled with saline) and needle enter the central vein by the chosen approach, maintaining suction on the syringe at all times.

Pass the Seldinger wire through the needle. This should pass freely and without any force into the vein. Watch for arrhythmias. Never pull the wire back through the needle once it has passed beyond the end of the bevel: it may shear off.

Use a scalpel blade to make a small nick in the skin. Hold the blade up and cut away from the wire.

If provided, pass the dilator over the wire into the vein. Then remove it, leaving the wire in situ.

Pass the cannula over the wire into the vein. Make sure that before you push the cannula forward the wire is visible at the proximal end. Hold on to the wire at all times, to prevent it being lost inside the patient!

For an average adult patient the central venous cannula does not need to be inserted more than 12–15 cm. Check markings on the cannula. Many are 20 cm long and do not need to be inserted up to the hub.

Draw back blood, flush all the lumens of the line with heparinized saline and lock off the three-way taps. At this point the patient can be levelled.

Suture the line into place using the anchorage devices provided and cover with an adhesive sterile dressing. 321

Attach a transducer and display the waveform on the monitor.

Dispose of your sharps and clear away your trolley.

Obtain CXR to verify position of the line and check for complications, including pneumothorax and haemothorax.

Document the procedure in the patient's notes.

**Position on Chest X-ray**

The catheter should lie along the long axis of the vessel and the tip should be in the superior vena cava (SVC) or at the junction of the SVC and right atrium but outside the pericardial reflection. The pericardium lies below the carina so ideally catheter tips should be at or above the level of the carina. Catheters below this level may perforate the heart and cause cardiac tamponade. Catheters placed via the left subclavian must not be allowed to lie with the tip abutting the wall of the superior vena cava. This may cause pain, perforation and accelerated thrombus formation. Either advance the catheter to lie in the long axis of the SVC or pull it back to lie in the brachiocephalic vein.

## COMMON PROBLEMS: CENTRAL VENOUS ACCESS

**Cannot Find the Vein**

Check position (ultrasound and/or landmarks) and try again. If unsuccessful do not persist with repeated passages of the needle in the hope of striking again. You may have misinterpreted the landmarks or the vein may be absent or occluded (e.g. with thrombus). Seek help.

## Aspirating Blood (needle in vein.) but Cannot Pass Wire

Check needle position by drawing back on the syringe; good flow is essential. Adjust the angle of incidence of the needle to the vein to improve flow. Tip the patient further head down to further extend the vein. Try rotating the needle through 180° and draw back again. Remember the wire must pass easily without force. If this doesn't work, repuncture the vein at a slightly different angle.

## Is it Arterial.

Occasionally, particularly if using a technique where the wire passes through the barrel of the syringe, it is difficult to know whether you have hit the artery or the vein. In this case it is important to avoid passing a large central venous catheter into the vessel until you are sure. Consider the following:

- Remove the syringe from the needle and observe for pulsatile flow.
- Connect a transducer directly to the needle in the vessel and look at the waveform.
- Pass the wire into the vessel and remove the needle. Pass an 18-gauge i.v. cannula over the wire into the vessel and remove the wire. Attach a transducer or manometer set directly to the cannula. When venous placement is confirmed, pass the wire back through the i.v. cannula and continue as before.

## Arterial Puncture

Needle only, then simply remove and press for 10 minutes. (Watch clock!) If large-bore cannula then action depends on circumstances. Usually can remove and press until bleeding stops. If severe coagulopathy, leave in situ and give platelets and FFP before removing. Seek advice and consider the need for surgical exploration and removal under direct vision.

## Complications

Complications of central venous cannulation depend in part on the route used.

The management of pneumothorax depends upon the size of the pneumothorax and the patient's condition, particularly whether he or she is ventilated or not. A small pneumothorax in an unventilated patient with good gas exchange may be observed, or aspirated using a small-bore cannula and syringe with three-way tap. Larger pneumothoraces, those that fail to resolve or those that cause any impairment of gas exchange and/or haemodynamics require a formal chest drain. Any significant haemothorax should be formally drained as soon as possible. Once blood has clotted in the chest, drainage is difficult. Seek cardiothoracic/surgical opinion. Bleeding around the puncture site can occasionally be a persistent problem. If this does not resolve with pressure, use a suture (5/0 Prolene) to tie a purse string around the puncture site. This usually stops the bleeding. Line colonization with bacteria and fungi is common and there is no evidence that changing lines on a regular basis (e.g. every 5–7 days) is of benefit.

## Changing Catheters Over a Wire

If new central venous catheters are required these should usually be placed at a clean site. Occasionally it may be necessary to change a catheter over a guide wire using an existing site. The technique is similar to that described above for placing any central venous catheter. The main problem is avoiding contamination of the new catheter.

Cut sutures on the old line before scrubbing.

Use universal precautions, aseptic technique, gown and gloves.

Clean and prep area.

Pass the wire down the central lumen of the old central venous catheter. (Make sure that the new wire is longer than the old CVP line.)

Remove the old catheter, leaving the wire in place, and send the tip of the old catheter for culture.

Clean the puncture site with antiseptic solution.

Use the wire to site the new line as required.

### Removing Central Venous Catheters

Removal of central venous catheters can precipitate air embolism, pneumothorax, haemothorax, embolization of thrombus and bacteraemia/sepsis. To remove central lines ensure that all drugs and infusions have been stopped or relocated to other lines. Lay the patient down to reduce the risk of air embolism and remove the line smoothly, applying pressure to the puncture site. Sit the patient up. If infection is suspected, send the tip of the line in a dry specimen pot for culture.

## LARGE-BORE INTRODUCER SHEATHS/DIALYSIS CATHETERS

### Indications

Introducer sheaths are available in a number of sizes for different applications, including insertion of pulmonary artery catheters and temporary pacing wires. In adults 7.5 or 8.5 Fr are generally used. They may be used as large-bore access for volume resuscitation. Smaller sheaths may be used for introducing specialized monitoring such as jugular bulb oximetery. Large-bore double lumen dialysis catheters are used for haemodialysis, haemofiltration, plasma exchange and rapid transfusion.

### Procedure

All these devices are inserted using a Seldinger technique and a large stiff dilator is used to dilate the initial needle track sufficiently to allow the large-bore catheter to be passed easily into the vessel. These dilators do not pass around a tight bend easily and can readily damage or perforate vessels. The left internal jugular vein is best avoided. Introducer sheaths can usually be sited safely at all other sites. Dialysis catheters may be best placed by the right internal jugular or femoral routes (particularly in patients with chronic renal failure, to preserve the venous drainage of the arm for subsequent AV fistulae formation).

Universal precautions. Aseptic technique, sterile gown and gloves.

Enter vein with needle, as for central venous line, and pass Seldinger wire.

Make small nick in the skin with a blade. Pass the sheath mounted on the introducer/dilator over the wire into the vein. The dilator is generally longer than needed and does not need to be passed right up to the hub. When the dilator has entered the vein, slide the sheath forward without advancing the dilator any further.

Remove wire and dilator. Draw back and flush with heparinized saline. (For dialysis catheters use heparin 1000 units/ml and flush to the volume of the catheter printed on the hub.)

When in situ and not in use the sheath port should be occluded with an obturator.

Get CXR to check position and complications.

The place of pulmonary artery catheters has been questioned recently and their use has diminished. They may be of value, however, in any condition in which haemodynamic instability or shock is unresponsive to fluid and inotrope therapy guided by conventional CVP measurement.

Use universal precautions.

Full aseptic technique. Sterile gowns and gloves.

Insert introducer sheath as above.

Position the patient flat before inserting the PA catheter. (This reduces the pulmonary artery pressures and reduces the risk of pulmonary artery rupture.)

Connect 3 three-way taps to the open ports, and flush lumens with heparinized saline.

Connect 1.5-ml syringe to the balloon port and test the balloon. (Check the size of the balloon before starting.)

Pass protective sleeve over PA catheter if provided.

Pass the proximal end of the catheter to an assistant who can connect a pressure transducer to the PA port (yellow) and flush the lumen. Then zero the transducer and check the signal on the monitor. Need to display trace on the monitor (scale 0–75 mmHg) continuously.

Calibrate fibreoptics if using a fibreoptic PA catheter.

Insert PA catheter into introducer sheath and pass to 20 cm. Note normal CVP trace.

Inflate balloon and advance catheter gently to right ventricle at approx. 30–40 cm. Advance further until the pulmonary artery is entered at approx. 40–50 cm.

Advance the catheter until pulmonary artery occlusion trace or wedge trace is observed, approx. 20 cm from RV (approx. 50–60 cm total). Deflate the balloon and see return of the PA trace.

Once the PA catheter is in position, perform a CXR

- Check the position of the catheter in the proximal pulmonary artery
- Exclude pneumothorax/haemothorax/knotting of the line.

While in use ensure that the PA pressure trace is displayed continuously on the bedside monitor so that inadvertent 'wedging' of the catheter can be recognized and the catheter pulled back to prevent pulmonary infarction.

## COMMON PROBLEMS: PULMONARY ARTERY CATHETERIZATION

### Catheter will not Take the Correct Path

This may be due to a dilated RV or low CO. Do not persist if unsuccessful:

- Remove completely, check direction of curvature of catheter and try again.
- To enter RV place patient head down and left side up.
- To enter PA place patient head up and supine.

### Catheter is'over wedged'

Always watch the pressure trace when wedging the catheter. If pressure rises then catheter is' over wedged'.

The catheter is too distal within the PA. There is a risk of pulmonary artery rupture. Deflate balloon, pull catheter back and try again.

### Catheter will not wedge

This may be because the catheter is curled up within the PA. Do not pass more than 20 cm without a change in trace. Pull back and try again.

In the presence of severe mitral regurgitation or pulmonary hypertension it may not be possible to obtain a satisfactory wedge trace and attempts may be associated with increased risk of PA rupture. Accept that the catheter will not wedge and use pulmonary diastolic pressure instead of PA occlusion pressure.

In low CO states there may be insufficient flow of blood in the pulmonary artery to advance the catheter when the balloon is inflated. Do not persist. Use PA diastolic as above.

### Complications

PA catheterization is not without risk and is certainly not a therapeutic manoeuvre in its own right! If patients are to benefit then regular collection and interpretation of haemodynamic and oxygen delivery variables, together with the appropriate therapeutic response, is required.

Most monitoring systems have a specific function key for use when measuring PAOP. These generally display the pulmonary artery pressure trace on a larger scale, allowing changes in the trace to be more easily observed and provide a cursor, which can be positioned to indicate the PAOP:

- Enter PAOP function on the monitor.
- Inflate the balloon and observe the wedge trace.
- Position cursor over the wedge trace' at the point corresponding to end expiration.

## THERMODILUTION MEASUREMENT OF CARDIAC OUTPUT

Pulmonary artery catheters incorporate a thermistor near the tip to allow thermodilution measurement of cardiac output. A volume of cold 5% dextrose solution (usually 10 ml) is injected through the central venous port of the PA catheter (in SVC or RA) and the temperature change in the PA is detected by the thermistor. The degree and the rate of temperature change is used to calculate cardiacoutput. (Some catheters incorporate a heated coil and fast reacting thermistor to allow continuous cardiac output measurement.)

Ensure that the correct cables are connected between the monitor and the PA catheter (one to the distal thermistor and one to measure the temperature of the injectate).

Enter cardiac output function on monitor.

Check that the correct computation constant is entered into the monitor. This depends upon the volume and temperature of the injectate and also the type of catheter used. The correct computation constant is found on the packaging information of the PA catheter.

Enter the patient's height and weight for calculation of body surface area (BSA).

Set the computer to measure cardiac output, and when prompted inject 10 ml of 5% dextrose into the right atrial (CVP) lumen of the PA catheter. Time the injection at the end of inspiration and inject as rapidly as possible.

Repeat the measurement. The individual cardiac output values obtained should not vary more than 5% from each other. Discard any inconsistent value and take the average reading for cardiac output. Having measured the cardiac output and PA occlusion pressure a range of haemodynamic variables can be calculated. This is generally performed by the monitoring system. In addition by measuring blood gases on blood drawn simultaneously from the pulmonary artery catheter (mixed venous) and an arterial line, oxygen delivery and consumption variables may be calculated.

## PERICARDIAL ASPIRATION

### Indications

Cardiac tamponade.

Large pericardial effusions.

To obtain diagnostic pericardial fluid. Small loculated effusions, not causing haemodynamic compromise and without diastolic collapse on echocardiogram, do not require pericardiocentesis. (See Pericardial effusion and cardiac tamponade, p. 90.)

### Procedure

Place patient supine with 20° of head-up tilt.

Establish i.v. access if not already present and monitor ECG.

Provide adequate sedation if necessary.

Full aseptic technique. Sterile gowns and gloves.

The point of needle insertion is immediately below and to the left of the xiphisternum, between the xiphisternum and the left costal margin. Infiltrate the skin and subcutaneous tissue with local anaesthetic.

Using a 10-ml syringe, advance the needle at 35° to the patient, beneath the costal margin and towards the left shoulder, aspirating continuously and observing the ECG.

Fluid (straw-coloured effusion or blood) is generally aspirated at a depth of 6–8 cm. Hold the needle stationary and pass the guide wire through the needle into the pericardial space.

Remove the needle, leaving the guide wire in situ and then pass the catheter over the wire into the pericardial space. Attach a three-way tap.

Use a 50-ml syringe to aspirate pericardial effusion or attach to a closed drainage system such as a vacuum bottle. Aspiration should produce immediate haemodynamic improvement.

Suture the drain in place.

### Complications

Performed carefully, complications are few. They include pneumothorax, ventricular tachycardia, myocardial puncture and damage to the coronary arteries. A repeat CXR and echocardiogram should be performed after the procedure to confirm adequate placement and drainage and to identify any problems. Insertion of a pericardial drain should only be considered a temporary measure. Seek general surgical or cardiothoracic surgical advice regarding repair of the underlying problem and/or creation of a pericardial window.

## DEFIBRILLATION AND DC CARDIOVERSION

### Indications

Treatment of any life-threatening 'shockable rhythm' according to advanced life support protocols.

### Procedure

Prior to 'elective' DC cardioversion, consider the need for anticoagulation (usually unnecessary except in chronic dysrhythmias).

Check the patient is adequately sedated/anaesthetized. This may require supplementation of sedation and analgesia in a ventilated patient with a small bolus dose of midazolam, opioid or other similar agent. Conscious patients will require anaesthesia, usually with a cardiostable drug such as etomidate.

Place conducting gel pads over the patient's apex and sternum,

Select the appropriate mode (asynchronous or synchronous) and select required energy levels (see relevant algorithms) before removing the paddles from the defibrillator.

Take paddles from the defibrillator and place immediately on to gel pads on the patient. Only charge the paddles once they are in contact with the patient.

Before charging paddles give an 'all clear' warning to ensure that no-one is touching the patient and check that everyone is clear.

Before delivering the shock, give a second all clear warning; check that everyone is clear and that any oxygen source is temporarily removed from the patient. Ensure that you yourself are not inadvertently in contact with the patient.

Deliver shock.

After delivery of the shock, several seconds may pass before monitors yield an ECG trace. Keep paddles in contact with the patient if you may wish to deliver a further shock, or return them to the safe position on the defibrillator.

If normal rhythm is not restored seek expert help. Consider:

- Higher energy shock.
- Alternative paddle position (e.g. cardiac long axis, anteroposterior).
- Use of antidysrhythmic drug before repeat attempts.

- Many patients on ICU develop atrial fibrillation that does not return to sinus rhythm for more than a very short period after DC cardioversion, until their underlying condition has improved.

## INTUBATION OF THE TRACHEA

This is covered at greater length in standard anaesthesia texts; however, there are some aspects of tracheal intubation of particular relevance to patients in intensive care.

### Indications

These fall broadly into three groups:

- Relieving airway obstruction, protection of the airway from aspiration and facilitation of artificial ventilation of the lungs.
- Patients requiring intubation in ICU frequently have limited physiological reserve and are liable to haemodynamic collapse.
- Drugs used to facilitate intubation must therefore be used judiciously.

In some cases patients may already have a markedly obtunded conscious level and small doses of benzodiazepines (e.g. diazepam 5–10 mg) may be all that is required. In other patients low doses of i.v. a naesthetic agents may be appropriate (e.g. propofol 1–2 mg/kg or etomidate 0.1–0.2 mg/kg); however, these may be associated with cardiovascular collapse.

Muscle relaxants will usually be required to facilitate intubation. Suxamethonium (1–2 mg/kg) is rapid in onset and relatively shortacting in most patients. It is the drug of choice for rapid sequence induction. It has a number of side effects, however, which limit its use. Atracurium (0.5 mg/kg) is an alternative but is slower in onset and has a longer duration of action.

**Procedure**

Preoxygenate the patient. Administer 100% oxygen using a tight-fitting face mask for a period of 3–4 minutes prior to administering any drugs or attempting intubation, if possible. This will wash out nitrogen and fill the functional residual capacity with oxygen, thereby providing an oxygen reservoir and increasing the safety margin in the event of difficulties.

Check the head is in the 'sniffing the morning air' position (neck flexed, atlantoaxial joint extended, one firm pillow).

If the patient might have a full stomach, ask your assistant to apply cricoid pressure; if the neck is supported from behind and the cricoid firmly gripped, downward pressure prevents any passive regurgitation. If possible, avoid inflating the lungs with the face mask and self-inflating bag until the tube is in place, as blowing air into the stomach may increase the risks of regurgitation.

Give sedative anaesthetic and muscle relaxant as appropriate.

Hold the laryngoscope in the left hand (size 3 or 4 Macintosh scopes are most commonly used). Slide the scope into the right of the mouth, sweeping the tongue into the groove in the blade, under it and to the left. As you advance the laryngoscope blade over the base of the tongue, the epiglottis pops into sight. With the blade between the epiglottis and the base of the tongue (vallecula), apply traction in the line of the laryngoscope handle, gently drawing the epiglottis forward and exposing the V-shaped glottis behind.

Pass the endotracheal tube between the vocal cords so that the cuff is just distal to them. There is usually a mark on the endotracheal tube above the cuff, which when placed at the level of the cords indicates the correct position of the tube.

If you can visualize the vocal cords but are having difficulty passing the endotracheal tube into the larynx, pass a gum elastic bougie or airway exchange catheter into the larynx and then try passing a lubricated endotracheal tube over this.

Inflate the cuff while ventilating through the endotracheal tube with the self-inflating bag until any gas leak just disappears.

Verify correct positioning of the tube by observation of chest movement, auscultation and if possible by capnography. Secure it, and attach to the ventilator via a suitable catheter mount. Recheck the tube position and chest movement.

Check the cuff pressure with a standard pressure gauge to reduce the risks of laryngeal mucosal injury.

Pass a nasogastric tube if this is not already in situ.

Obtain a CXR to confirm tube position. Check if the tube is too short, too long. Check for lobar collapse, pneumothorax, etc.

## Complications

Potential complications of endotracheal intubation are :

- The commonest and most immediately life-threatening complication is oesophageal intubation.
- If in doubt, remove the tube, ventilate by face mask, and start again. Nasal intubation may provoke epistaxis or predispose to mucosal injury (e.g. submucosal positioning of the tube).
- In the longer term, nasal intubation may occlude the maxillary antrum and give rise to sinusitis.
- It is nevertheless better tolerated than oral intubation, particularly during weaning from ventilation.

- Long-term complications include erosion and stenosis of local tissues, particularly of the larynx and trachea.
- This may present as airway obstruction and stridor after extubation.

## EXTUBATION OF THE TRACHEA

Before you consider extubation, the patient should be breathing spontaneously with a satisfactory respiratory pattern and acceptable blood gases. The patient should have an appropriate conscious level and airway reflexes and not be requiring repeated airway suctioning.

Check a suitable system for providing humidified oxygen by face mask is available, and you have everything necessary for reintubation.

Explain to the patient what you are going to do, then aspirate any secretions from the posterior pharynx.

Insert a wide-bore suction catheter through the endotracheal tube.

Deflate the cuff, and simultaneously aspirate through the suction catheter as you withdraw the endotracheal tube. This ensures that any secretions that have collected above the cuff are removed.

Finally, fit a face mask and encourage the patient to cough out any further secretions.

Observe the patient closely for signs of respiratory inadequacy or distress developing over the next few hours.

## INSERTION OF LARYNGEAL MASK

In the event of being unable to intubate a patient it is vital that oxygenation is maintained. Laryngeal masks are relatively simple to use, provide a clear airway and effectively free the operator's hands. Laryngeal masks come in a range of sizes for all ages. Size 3 is suitable for average adult females and size 4 for average adult males.

Maintain oxygenation by bag and mask.

Deflate the cuff of the laryngeal mask.

Lubricate with aqueous gel.

Pass into the mouth and push back over the tongue into the oropharynx until the laryngeal mask fits naturally in the posterior pharynx.

Inflate the cuff with 20–30 ml of air.

Attach breathing circuit.

Gently ventilate the patient with 100% oxygen and check for chest movement and end-tidal $CO_2$.

Seek senior help to secure airway by endotracheal intubation.

## PERCUTANEOUS TRACHEOSTOMY

In recent years tracheostomy has become a common procedure on the ICU. Traditionally, tracheostomy was only performed after patients had been intubated for about 10–14 days because of fear of laryngeal and subglottic injury resulting from continued intubation. The advent of percutaneous techniques has allowed tracheostomy to be performed safely and easily at the bedside without the use of specialized surgical instruments, lighting or diathermy. As a result, many units now perform tracheostomy earlier.

## ADVANTAGES OF TRACHEOSTOMY

These include:

- More comfortable than naso-/orotracheal tubes, which allows significant reductions in muscle relaxants, sedative and analgesic drugs. This promotes return of GI tract function.
- Patients easily switched from IPPV/assist modes/ CPAP/T-piece without the need for extubation and reintubation.
- Easier clearance of tracheal secretions by suction.

- Speech is possible with cuff deflation or speaking tube.
- There may be a lower risk of airway problems after prolonged tracheostomy than after prolonged translaryngeal intubation. Narrowing and scarring of the major airways is a potential risk in both situations.

## Indications

Actual or impending airway obstruction. Tracheostomy should be considered early, before progressive swelling makes reintubation in the event of tube blockage or dislodgement potentially impossible.

Known difficult intubation.

The need for prolonged IPPV.

Aid to weaning.

Inability of patients to protect or maintain their own airway in the longer term, e.g. severe brain injury, bulbar palsy.

## Procedure

Explain to the patient (and relatives) what you are going to do. Get written or verbal consent. Check the patient's coagulation status. Position the patient flat with the head and neck extended over a pillow. The majority of patients are already intubated and ventilated and are given either an intravenous or volatile anaesthetic. This is supplemented by infiltration of the surgical area with 10 ml of local anaesthetic plus adrenaline (epinephrine), which helps reduces skin edge bleeding.

A bronchoscope can be passed into the larynx during the procedure (through the endotracheal tube or laryngeal mask). This allows the operator to visualize the needle puncture of the trachea and the correct placement of guide wire, dilator and tracheostomy tube. A camera system and monitor make this much easier.

## Anaesthetist

Ensure appropriate monitoring and anaesthetize patient with inhalational or intravenous technique as appropriate. Beware of relying solely on intermittent bolus of propofol, as there is a risk of 'awareness'. A muscle relaxant is usually required.

Suction trachea and oropharynx.

Ventilate with 100% oxygen throughout the procedure.

When the operator is ready, withdraw the endotracheal tube under direct vision using a laryngoscope, until the cuff is visible at the laryngeal inlet. This prevents the endotracheal tube being transfixed by the operator's needle when the trachea is punctured.

Care must be taken not to lose the airway when the tube is withdrawn. Consider passing a gum elastic bougie or airway exchange catheter down the tube prior to withdrawal to ensure the tube can be replaced if it is pulled back too far. (Equipment must be available to reintubate the patient in case of difficulty.)

An alternative approach is to remove the endotracheal tube altogether and to use a laryngeal mask to maintain ventilation and oxygenation.

If a bronchoscope is to be used, pass this down the endotracheal tube or laryngeal mask and into the larynx so that the operator has a view of the trachea at the level at which needle puncture will occur.

Maintain ventilation until the procedure is complete and then pass the catheter mount to the operator to attach to the tracheostomy tube.

## Operator

Tracheostomy may be safely performed through the cricothyroid membrane or in the subcricoid region. In the UK it is recommended that the tracheostomy stoma should be between the 2nd and 4th tracheal rings. At higher levels there may be an increased risk of laryngeal/tracheal stenosis, which may ultimately necessitate tracheal resection. At lower levels there is an increased risk of haemorrhage from major vessels in the thoracic inlet. There are a number of different percutaneous tracheostomy kits available. Most require that the trachea is punctured by a needle and a guide wire passed through the needle into the lumen of the trachea. This is then used to guide a tracheal dilator, which creates the tracheostomy, allowing the insertion of a tracheostomy tube. The following notes are a guide only, the exact details of the method of insertion will depend upon the system used.

Check that all necessary equipment is available and prepared.

Position patient flat with the neck extended over a pillow.

Examine the neck and ascertain the position of the trachea. Look for anatomical abnormalities, large veins or palpable arterial pulsation. (Ultrasound gives good images of deeper vessels that may be at risk during the procedure.)

Clean the skin.

Palpate the cricothyroid membrane and sternal notch. Infiltrate the skin with 1% lidocaine (lignocaine) and adrenaline (epinephrine), midway between the two.

Make a 2-cm superficial incision horizontally across the midline.

Use blunt forceps and a finger to dissect the pretracheal tissue until you can feel the tracheal rings and identify the level. If necessary, tie off the anterior jugular veins, which occasionally bleed.

Ask the anaesthetist to withdraw the endotracheal tube until the tip is just within the larynx.

Puncture the trachea with the introducer needle below the level of the first tracheal ring and in the midline. Using a saline-filled syringe, confirm the position of the needle by aspiration of air/mucus from the trachea. A bronchoscope passed through the endotracheal tube can also be used to confirm the correct position of the needle tip within the tracheal lumen.

Pass the guide wire through the needle into the trachea and remove the needle.

Dilate the trachea according to the manufacturer's instructions supplied with the tracheostomy kit used and insert the tracheostomy tube, again according to instructions.

Remove the introducer and guide wire.

Suck out any blood from the trachea. Blood clot in the airway may produce total airway obstruction or act as a ball valve, allowing gas in but not out.

Inflate the cuff and ventilate the patient through the tracheostomy.

Correct placement of the tube may be confirmed by bronchoscopy or capnography. Check that chest expansion is symmetrical and that there are bilateral breath sounds, and that oxygen saturations are maintained.

Tie the tracheostomy tube in place using tracheostomy tapes. In addition, it is advisable to place two stay sutures through the wings of the tracheostomy tube to prevent early accidental decannulation.

Obtain a chest X-ray to confirm position and exclude any complications.

## COMMON PROBLEMS DURING PERCUTANEOUS TRACHEOSTOMY

### Bleeding

Heavy bleeding from the wound may sometimes occur, particularly if an anterior jugular vein is damaged. If possible place a clip on the bleeding vessel and tie off. Otherwise pack the wound with gauze, apply pressure and wait. If you are near the end of the procedure insert the tracheostomy tube, as this will often tamponade the bleeding. If bleeding does not stop, consider removing the tracheostomy tube (reintubate the patient via the oral route and pass the endotracheal tube beyond the stoma), pack the wound and seek surgical assistance.

### Difficulty Ventilating the Patient

This usually means that the tracheostomy tube has been misplaced. Do not persist as this may produce a tension pneumothorax! Remove the tracheostomy tube and reintubate the patient by the oral (nasal) route.

### Complications

Air emphysema is common but, unless accompanied by a pneumothorax, is usually unimportant and will resolve over time. Pneumothorax is generally the result of attempting to ventilate the patient through a misplaced tube, resulting in air tracking down into the mediastinum and pleural cavities.

### Care of the Patient with a Tracheostomy

Patients with tracheostomy tubes should receive adequate humidification of inspired gases to prevent drying, and regular suction to remove secretions. Spare tracheostomy tubes of the same size and one size smaller should be kept at the bedside, together with a pair of tracheal dilators.

### Choice of Tracheostomy Tubes

A wide range of tracheostomy tubes in different lengths and sizes is available. Tubes with adjustable flanges are available to cater for patients in whom standard tubes are not suitable (e.g. those with very fat necks, goitres, etc.). Tubes with removable inner sleeves are useful for preventing build-up of secretions on the inner surface of the tube. In long-term patients, fenestrated or valved tubes, which allow speaking, may be useful.

### Changing Tracheostomy Tubes

Tracheostomy tubes can be changed at any time if necessary, but it is more difficult if the tract is not well established. Give the patient 100% oxygen and position as for performing a tracheostomy. Pass a large-bore suction catheter (with the end cut off) or gum elastic bougie through the old tracheostomy tube before removing it and use this as a guide to insert the new tube. Facilities for ventilating the patient with a bag and mask and for reintubation should be available in case of difficulty.

### Decannulations

When the patient's condition has improved, the question of when to remove the tracheostomy tube inevitably arises. Consideration should be given to the following:

- Respiratory effort
- Volume of tracheal secretions and ability to cough
- Laryngeal competence and ability to swallow pharyngeal secretions
- General condition and strength Ï% conscious level.

There is no difficulty in a trial of decannulation, providing the tract is well formed (5–7 days after insertion). It is not routine practice to stitch up stomas: they are usually left to granulate on their own. A simple occlusive dressing should be applied over the stoma. Ideally, patients should be seen in an ICU follow-up clinic. If tracheal stenosis or other problems develop, appropriate referral can be made.

## CRICOTHYROIDOTOMY/MINITRACHEOSTOMY

Cricothyroidotomy is a life-saving procedure used to provide emergency access to the airway (e.g. following obstruction of the upper airway) when measures such as bag and mask ventilation and tracheal intubation have failed. It involves the insertion of a small tube through the cricothyroid membrane, through which oxygen/ventilation can be provided until a definitive airway is obtained. Minitracheostomy is a term used to describe the insertion of a similar small-bore non-cuffed tube through the cricothyroid membrane (4 mm internal diameter), principally to aid the clearance of secretions. The passage of suction catheters stimulates coughing and allows secretions to be aspirated. As a short-term measure these devices may help to prevent the need for naso-/orotracheal intubation and assisted ventilation. The small size of the tube limits its value and the use of minitracheostomy has declined in recent years. Both cricothyroidotomy and minitracheostomy kits are commercially available. The technique for the insertion of each is essentially the same.

**Procedure**

Explain to the patient what you are going to do. Get written or verbal consent if appropriate. Check the patient's coagulation status. Position the patient comfortably with the head and neck extended over a pillow. Then:

- Palpate anatomy to identify the cricothyroid membrane.

  Clean the neck with antiseptic solution.

- Infiltrate over the cricothyroid membrane with 2–3 ml of local anaesthetic.
- Warn the patient that you are going to make him or her cough and perform cricothyroid puncture with a green 21-gauge needle.
- Aspirate air to confirm the tracheal position of the needle and rapidly inject 2 ml of lidocaine (lignocaine). Wait for coughing to subside.
- Perform a superficial skin incision.
- Pass the introducing needle into the trachea and aspirate air.
- Pass the guide wire through the needle and then remove the needle.
- Pass the introducer over the guide wire and then slide the cricothyroidotomy/minitracheostomy tube

off the introducer. Remove the introducer and guide wire together, leaving the cricothyroidotomy/minitracheostomy in place. Suction to remove any blood.

- Obtain CXR to verify the position.

### Complications

The complications of minitracheostomy are the same as for formal tracheostomy. Misplacement and bleeding are particular problems.

## BRONCHOSCOPY

Flexible fibreoptic bronchoscopy is a useful diagnostic and therapeutic tool in the ICU. In this situation it is usually performed on patients who have access to their airway via an endotracheal tube or tracheostomy.

### Indications

Fibreoptic intubation.

Removal of secretions (associated with areas of collapse on CXR).

Retrieval of sputum samples for microbiology.

Bronchoalveolar lavage (see below).

Assessment of airway injury and burns.

Biopsy of tumours and lung tissue.

Assessment of endotracheal tube position.

To guide operator during tracheostomy (see above).

### Contraindications

These are relative. Patients with high airway pressures, critical oxygenation, cardiovascular instability or raised intracranial pressure may not tolerate bronchoscopy.

### Preparation

The bronchoscope should be leak-tested and sterilized before use. This generally takes about 20 minutes. Most hospitals will have automatic washers for this.

### Procedure

Before commencing the procedure, check that the size of the patient's endotracheal tube is adequate to allow bronchoscopy. Tubes smaller than 8 mm internal diameter may be significantly occluded by the bronchoscope, making ventilation and oxygenation of the patient difficult.

Attach the swivel connector to the patient's endotracheal or tracheostomy tube.

Ventilate the patient on 100% oxygen prior to and during the bronchoscopy.

Adequately sedate the patient and then give a small dose of muscle relaxant (such as atracurium) to prevent the patient biting or coughing on the bronchoscope. Instil 3–5 ml of local anaesthetic (e.g. 1% lidocaine (lignocaine)) down the trachea. It is sensible to have an assistant to look after patient sedation and ventilation while you perform the bronchoscopy.

Bronchoscopy should be a clean procedure to avoid contaminating the patient's airway.

Lubricate the scope with a small amount of lubricant jelly. Avoid getting it over the lens.

Pass the bronchoscope through the bung on the swivel connector and into the endotracheal or tracheostomy tube. Continue forward under direct vision.

Pass the scope forward to the carina. Then explore each side of the bronchial tree in turn. Identify and enter each lobar and segmental bronchus. Take note of any abnormal anatomy and remove any secretions.

If there are thick secretions that cannot be sucked up the scope, try instilling 10–20 ml of sterile saline down the suction port of the bronchoscope. This may help to loosen them. Large plugs and blood clots may be dragged out on the end of the scope.

To obtain microbiology specimens place a sputum trap in between the bronchoscope and the wall suction. Use a separate trap for each side. Be careful to keep the sputum trap upright to prevent the secretions disappearing down the suction tubing. Also remove sputum traps before removing the scope from the patient to prevent specimens being contaminated with upper airway flora.

Bronchial biopsy should not be performed by trainees in intensive care. Seek help.

Following bronchoscopy, perform a CXR to exclude pneumothorax and look for improvement in lung expansion where large sputum plugs have been removed.

Ensure the scope is washed and sterilized according to your hospital policy.

## BRONCHOALVEOLAR LAVAGE

Bronchoalveolar lavage (BAL) is a technique for obtaining microbiology specimens from low in the respiratory tree, avoiding contamination of samples with upper respiratory tract flora. It may be performed during bronchoscopy or using specially designed BAL catheters.

### Indications

BAL may be used to obtain specimens in any patient with pneumonia. It is of particular value in investigating pneumonia in the immunocompromised patient. In addition to conventional pathogens such as *Streptococcus pneumoniae* and *Haemophilus influenzae*, other likely pathogens in these patients are *Pneumocystis carinii*, either alone or with a copathogen, *Mycobacterium* species including tuberculosis, cytomegalovirus and fungi.

Discuss the clinical situation with a microbiologist before performing the BAL. He or she will advise on appropriate specimens and tests.

## BAL During Bronchoscopy

This has the advantage that the operator can be highly selective in the area for lavage in the case of localized disease. It is, however, more invasive and operator-dependent.

During bronchoscopy (see above) the bronchoscope is passed into a subsegmental bronchus until it wedges.

Up to 100 ml of saline is instilled down the suction channel.

This is then aspirated and collected into a series of sputum traps.

## BAL Using Catheter

BAL catheters consist of a protective outer sleeve and an inner suction catheter. The suction catheter can be connected via a three-way tap to suction and a syringe for instilling saline. This should be a clean procedure and you should wear apron, gloves and goggles.

Preoxygenate the patient with 100% oxygen.

Pass the catheter, with inner tube protected, into the airway, beyond the endotracheal tube.

Advance the inner protected suction catheter forwards until it meets resistance. Do not use undue force.

Perform BAL according to local protocol. Generally 80–100 ml of saline are instilled down the suction catheter, and then aspirated into 2 or 3 sputum traps. Not all the saline may be aspirated. This does not matter.

Withdraw the inner suction catheter into the protective sleeve before removing from the patient.

Having performed a BAL, telephone the laboratory and then send samples immediately with full diagnostic information and appropriate requests.

## CHEST DRAINAGE

### Indications

Chest drains are indicated for the drainage of air (pneumothorax), blood (haemothorax), fluid (pleural effusion), pus (empyema) and lymph (chylothorax) from the pleural cavity. In critically ill patients pleural fluid is a common finding on chest X-rays, CT scan and ultrasound. In most cases unless the effusion is large or ventilation is clearly compromised there is no need to drain this fluid. It will resolve as the patient's condition improves. Blood in the pleural cavity should be drained as soon as possible. Once it becomes clotted it will not drain readily and thoracotomy may be required to remove the clot and allow the lung to re-expand.

### Type of Drain

Chest drains are of two types. Traditionally large-bore tubes, particularly suitable for draining blood or pus, have been placed manually through an incision made in the chest wall directly into the pleural cavity. More recently, Seldinger versions have become available. Seldinger drains should only be used blindly to drain obvious large collections because of the risk that the introducer needle may damage the lung. For smaller collections, Seldinger drains should be placed under ultrasound guidance to reduce the risks of needle damage.

### Site of Drain

This is partly dictated by the position of the collection clinically and radiographically. In the case of long-standing collections, which may be loculated, ultrasound guidance may be helpful. In all other cases the drain should be sited in the 5th intercostal space, just anterior to the midaxillary line, and can be directed cephalad for air and caudally for fluid or blood. All drains should be placed immediately above the rib to avoid damage to the neurovascular bundle, which lies underneath.

**Procedure**

*Insertion of drain through thoracostomy*

Explain procedure to the patient.

Position the patient (supine with arm lifted, a pillow behind back).

Prepare a sterile field.

Infiltrate superficial structures down to rib with local anaesthetic.

Make a 2–4 cm incision.

Palpate through skin incision and perform blunt dissection down to rib and through pleura.

Push finger into pleural cavity and sweep around to ensure no viscera are adjacent.

Insert drain and direct into appropriate position.

Connect to underwater drain and confirm position by drainage of collection and respiratory swing.

Secure drain in position with suture. Purse-string sutures result in very unsightly scarring when chest drains are removed and are best avoided. Use mattress sutures to close the skin edges and a simple tie to hold in the drain.

Order a chest X-ray.

*Insertion of Seldinger Drains and Pigtail Catheters*

Explain procedure to the patient and position as before.

Ideally determine and mark the optimal position for drain site using ultrasound.

Prepare a sterile field.

Infiltrate superficial structures down to rib with local anaesthetic.

Advance needle through chest until blood/fluid/air aspirated.

Feed guide wire into pleural space.

Pass chest drain/pigtail catheter over guide wire.

For large drains attach underwater seal as above, for pigtail catheters aspirate and/or attach drainage bag.

Order a CXR.

## COMMON PROBLEMS DURING INSERTION OF CHEST DRAINS

### Lung will not Expand

Reassess diagnosis and position of tube.

Is tube 'swinging' or is it blocked/kinked. Is the effusion loculated.

Consider low-pressure suction (wall suction or pump 10–20 mmHg).

Increase tidal volume or add 10 cm of PEEP.

Consider need for surgical referral.

### Persistent Air Leak

Check the drain and reposition if necessary (it may have come out of the chest and be entraining room air). If air leak persists, attempt to minimize airway pressures.

In trauma patients, consider bronchoscopy to exclude airway rupture.

Wean patient onto spontaneous breathing modes.

If ventilated, ensure adequate sedation, analgesia and muscle relaxation.

Use pressure-controlled ventilation and reduce PEEP.

Accept a degree of hypercapnia.

Consider high frequency jet ventilation.

Consider thoracic surgical opinion.

### Indications for Urgent Thoracic Surgical Opinion

The combination of persistent air leak and non-compliant lungs (e.g. ARDS) may make adequate ventilation and gas exchange impossible. Urgent thoracic surgical opinion may be required.

### Removing Chest Drains

Chest drains can be removed when they are no longer needed. In practice, this means that if the clinical and CXR findings that required a chest drain have resolved, and the drain is no longer bubbling or draining fluid, it can be removed.

There is no need to clamp drains before removal.

Clean the site with antiseptic solution. Cut the retaining suture, remove the drain and occlude by pressing.

Close the wound with a suture. If this is already in situ it can be tied as the drain is removed to reduce any air entrainment.

Obtain a CXR.

## PASSING A NASOGASTRIC TUBE

All patients in the ICU who require ventilation require a nasogastric tube, initially at least, to ensure gastric drainage and early enteral feeding.

### Procedure

Explain to the patient what you are going to do, even if he or she is apparently unconscious. Position the patient supine with head neutral.

Lubricate the NG tube and, keeping alignment with the long axis of the patient, introduce through the nose. Do not force. If resistance is met, try the other side.

If the patient is co-operative ask the patient to swallow the tip of the tube when he or she feels it in the back of the throat. In unconscious patients the tube may pass directly into the oesophagus but often coils up in the mouth.

In this case, use a laryngoscope to examine the pharynx and pass the tube manually into the oesophagus using a pair of Magill forceps. (Be careful not to traumatize the uvula and pharyngeal mucosa.)

Confirm the position of the NG tube in the stomach by aspiration of gastric contents (turns litmus paper red), auscultation (gurgling when air blown into tube) or by CXR. The presence of a cuffed endotracheal or tracheostomy tube does not prevent feeding tubes entering the lung.

Secure the NG tube in position with adhesive tape.

### Nasojejunal Feeding Tubes

Nasojejunal feeding tubes are fine-bore soft tubes designed for long-term use. They are usually provided with the feeding tube mounted on a wire insert, which stiffens the tube during placement and allows X-ray determination of position. This is removed once the tube is in place. The main difficulty in passing nasojejunal feeding tubes is getting them to pass through the pylorus. The simplest approach is to pass a reasonable length of tube into the stomach (as for NG tube above) and leave for a few hours before getting an abdominal X-ray. Some tubes will simply migrate into the duodenum/jejunum. Alternatively, jejunal tubes can be placed using X-ray screening, ultrasound or endoscopic guidance. Seek advice.

## PASSING A SENGSTAKEN-BLAKEMORE TUBE

A number of tubes have been designed to apply pressure to oesophageal varices in order to compress the vessels and reduce bleeding while the patient is resuscitated and definitive treatment carried out. The Sengstaken-Blakemore tube has three lumens. Two are used to inflate balloons, one in the stomach and the other in the oesophagus, while the third is used to aspirate gastric contents.

**Procedure**

Read instructions for the specific device you are using.

Explain to the patient what you are going to do.

Position the patient comfortably. Left lateral is best if the patient is vomiting.

Check the patency of the tube lumens and integrity of the balloons.

Pass the tube orally into the oesophagus and down into the stomach. (Local anaesthetic spray to the pharynx may make this more tolerable in the awake patient.) Insert the tube to at least 30 cm.

Inflate the gastric balloon with 250 ml of saline. You should not feel any resistance.

Pull the tube backwards gently until resistance is felt as the gastric balloon meets the gastro-oesophageal junction.

Inflate the oesophageal balloon with air or saline (approximately 100 ml). The pressure in the oesophageal balloon can be measured using a sphygmomanometer and should be 25–35 mmHg. Chest pain, respiratory difficulty and cardiac arrhythmias may occur during inflation of the balloon.

Apply traction to the tube by tying a piece of string to the end and suspending a 500-ml bag of fluid over a fulcrum. Traction should be released at regular intervals to prevent pressure necrosis of the gastro-oesophageal junction.

The position of the tube should be checked by CXR. The point where the tube exits the mouth should be marked in order to detect subsequent migration. Check the pressure in the oesophageal balloon regularly.

### Removing the Tube

After 24 hours the traction should be removed and the oesophageal balloon deflated to assess for bleeding. If bleeding recurs, the balloon can be reinflated for a further period of 24 hours; however, the need for surgery becomes increasingly likely. If there is no bleeding the tube is generally left in situ deflated for 24 hours in case bleeding recurs. After this time the tube can be removed.

## TURNING A PATIENT PRONE

Patients may be turned prone when oxygenation is critical despite ventilation and high inspired oxygen concentrations. Turning large adult patients prone can be hazardous both for the staff and the patient. Where possible, hoists or other aids to handling patients should be used. The nursing staff will advise on the best approach. In general terms, whatever approach to physically turning the patient is adopted, there must be adequate numbers of staff available to ensure patient safety, and security of airway, vascular cannulae and drains, etc.

Temporarily discontinue all non-essential drug and fluid infusions.

Ensure that all lines and monitoring cables are positioned such that they will not be trapped under the patient when he or she is turned.

Remove ECG electrodes from the patient's front and replace on the back.

Designate specific individuals to be responsible for maintaining the security of the endotracheal tube, vascular access and lines. Designate other individuals to turn the patient.

Position pillows so that they will be under the patient's chest and pelvis when the patient is prone. Alternatively, position them afterwards. They are to ensure that the abdomen is not compressed, which can impair venous return and CO.

When everyone is ready, use the commands 'ready, steady, move'. Turn the patient on 'move'.

Ensure the patient is comfortably positioned and that there is no pressure on the tip of the nose, eyes or any peripheral nerves. The arms should be positioned towards the patient's head (not unduly extended) to ensure there is no tension on the brachial plexus.

Re-establish any monitoring or drugs and fluid infusions that were previously discontinued.

## TRANSPORTING CRITICALLY ILL PATIENTS

Critically ill patients in intensive care often require transport either within the hospital (for example for investigations or surgery), or between hospitals (for example for specialist care). You are therefore likely to be involved in transporting a patient at some stage, even if only within your own hospital.

The standards of care during transport, whether intrahospital or interhospital, should be the same as that provided within the ICU. Before moving the patient, it is important that the patient is fully resuscitated and stable. If there is any doubt regarding the adequacy of resuscitation, this should be addressed before transfer. The general principles are as follows:

- Full monitoring should be continued. This should include blood pressure monitoring (preferably invasive), ECG, oxygen saturation, and end-tidal CO2 for intubated/ventilated patients. If a PA catheter is in situ the pressure trace must be displayed, or the catheter should be pulled back into the SVC to prevent inadvertent pulmonary artery occlusion.
- Ensure that the airway is secure; this usually means endotracheal intubation.

- Ensure adequate supplies of oxygen to complete the transfer. In case the supply fails, an alternative means of ventilating the patient should be available. This should be a self-inflating bag, rather than an anaesthetic breathing circuit.
- Ensure that a portable suction unit is available.
- Ensure adequate intravenous access, usually at least two secure intravenous cannulae.
- Discontinue non-essential drug infusions. Ensure that essential infusions are delivered using syringe pumps with fully charged batteries.
- Ensure any drugs or resuscitation equipment that you are likely to need during the transfer are available. During the transfer you should be accompanied by an intensive care nurse or an operating department assistant. The transfer should be fully documented, including a record of pulse, blood pressure, ventilation and other vital signs. Departure and arrival times should be notified to the receiving hospital sufficiently in advance to enable suitable preparation to be made.

# Chapter 7

# Caring of Cardiac Patient

## INTRODUCTION

Ischemic heart disease results from an inadequate level of coronary blood flow to meet myocardial oxygen demand. The heart extracts oxygen nearly maximally at baseline, and thus increases in demand must be met by commensurate increases in coronary blood flow. Myocardial infarction (MI) occurs when prolonged ischemia causes myocardial necrosis.

Myocardial ischemia is associated almost immediately with failure of contraction. Although this can result in part from myocardial necrosis, areas of nonfunctional but viable myocardium can also cause or contribute to the development of systolic dysfunction. This reversibly dysfunctional myocardium comes under two main categories: stunning and hibernation. Myocardium reperfused after ischemia may exhibit profound contractile dysfunction despite restoration of normal blood flow, but may recover eventually; this transient postischemic dysfunction is termed "stunning". Hibernating myocardium is a state of persistently impaired myocardial function at rest due to severely reduced coronary blood flow, and can be viewed as a response that reduces myocardial contractile function in an area of hypoperfusion so as to restore equilibrium between flow and function, thus minimizing the potential for ischemia or necrosis. Both stunned and hibernating myocardium have contractile reserve, and function of both may improve with time and/ or revascularization.

## PATHOGENESIS

Myocardial infarction is usually due to thrombus formation within a coronary artery, most often resulting from rupture of an atherosclerotic plaque. Classification of infarctions into those which are transmural and those which are nontransmural has been largely abandoned due to the recognition that electrocardiographic criteria are neither sensitive nor specific to make this distinction. Infarctions can be usually into Q-wave infarctions, which are usually transmural and most often result from total coronary occlusion, and non-Q-wave infarctions, which are usually subendocardial and result from subtotal coronary occlusion. More recently, MI has been divided based on the presence of ST-segment elevation at presentation. This classification is useful clinically because patients with ST-elevation MI are eligible for thrombolytic therapy, and patients with non-ST elevation MI are not.

## DISTRIBUTIONS OF THE MAJOR CORONARY ARTERIES

The left anterior descending coronary artery (LAD) supplies the anterior left ventricle, anterior septum and usually the left ventricular apex; the LAD has septal and diagonal branches. Anterior infarction is seen in electrocardiographic (ECG) leads V1 to V5. The right coronary artery (RCA) supplies the inferior left ventricular wall, usually the inferior septum, most of the right ventricle, and the sinus node. The RCA is dominant (that is, it gives rise to a posterior descending artery and so supplies left ventricular myocardium in the inferior septal region) in 80% of patients. Inferior infarction is seen in ECG leads II, III, and aVF. The circumflex coronary artery runs in the atrioventricular (A-V) groove; obtuse marginal (OM) branches supply the lateral and posterolateral left ventricle. Lateral infarction is seen in ECG leads I, aVL, V5, and V6.

## DIAGNOSIS OF ACUTE INFARCTION

The diagnosis of acute MI is made on the basis of a compatible clinical presentation, ECG changes, and a rise and fall in enzymes indicative of myocardial damage. The differential diagnosis of acute infarction includes dissecting aortic aneurysm, pericarditis, pulmonary processes such as pulmonary embolism, pneumonia, and pneumothorax, gastrointestinal processes such as esophageal or peptic ulcer disease and cholecystitis, and costochondritis.

The classic electrocardiographic feature of acute infarction is ST segment elevation, followed by T-wave inversion and ultimate development of Q waves. The diagnosis can be limited in the presence of pre-existing left bundle-branch block (LBBB) or permanent pacemaker. Nonetheless, new LBBB with a compatible clinical presentation should be treated as acute MI and treated accordingly. True posterior MI, which usually accompanies inferior infarction, can be subtle; hallmarks include prominent R waves, tall upright T waves, and depressed ST segments in leads V1 and V2. The clinician must also be careful not to be fooled by ECG "imposters" of acute infarction, which include pericarditis, J-point elevation, Wolff-Parkinson-White syndrome, and hypertrophic cardiomyopathy.

The classic biochemical marker of acute MI is elevation of creatine phosphokinase (CPK) levels. The CPK MB isoenzyme is found primarily in cardiac muscle, and only small amounts are present in skeletal muscle and brain. CPK peaks during the first 24 hrs and then decreases rapidly. Lactate dehydrogenase (LDH) levels peak at 72 to 96 hrs and may be used to detect recent infarction, which is associated with an increase in the LDH1 isoenzyme.

Elevations in troponin T and troponin I are more specific biochemical markers of cardiac muscle damage. Their use is becoming more widespread, and has superceded use of CPK MB in many settings. Troponins are more sensitive and specific for the detection of myocardial damage, and troponin elevation in patients without ST elevation (or in fact, without elevation of CPK-MB) identifies a subpopulation at increased risk for complications. Troponins may not be elevated until 6 hrs after an acute event, and once elevated, remain high for days to weeks, limiting their utility to detect late reinfarction.

## THROMBOLYTIC THERAPY FOR ACUTE MYOCARDIAL INFARCTION

Early reperfusion of an occluded coronary artery is indicated for all eligible candidates. Thrombolytic therapy has been proven to decrease mortality in patients with ST-segment elevation; patients treated early derive the most benefit. Indications and contraindications for thrombolytic therapy are listed below. Contraindications can be regarded as absolute or relative.

### Indications

- Symptoms consistent with acute myocardial infarction.
- ECG showing 1-mm (0.1 mV) ST elevation in at least two contiguous leads, or new LBBB.
- Presentation within 12 hrs of symptom onset.
- Absence of contraindications.

### Contraindications

*Absolute*

- Active internal bleeding
- Intracranial neoplasm, aneurysm, or A-V malformation

- Stroke or neurosurgery within 6 wks
- Trauma or major surgery within 2 wks which could be a potential source of serious rebleeding
- Aortic dissection

*Relative*

- Prolonged (>10 mins) or clearly traumatic cardiopulmonary resuscitation
- Severe uncontrolled hypertension (>200/110 mm Hg)
- Trauma or major surgery within 6 wks (but more than 2 wks)
- Pre-existing coagulopathy
- Active peptic ulcer
- Infective endocarditis
- Pregnancy
- Chronic severe hypertension (Could be an absolute contraindication in low-risk patients with MI)

## THROMBOLYTIC AGENTS

Streptokinase (SK) is a single-chain protein produced by -hemolytic streptococci, which produces a systemic lytic state for about 24 hrs. SK is given as a 1.5 million-unit iv infusion over 1 hr. Hypotension with infusion usually responds to fluids and a decreased infusion rate, but allergic reactions are possible. Hemorrhagic complications are the most feared side-effect, with a rate of intracranial hemorrhage of approximately 0.5%.

Tissue plasminogen activator (t-PA) is a recombinant protein that is more fibrin-selective than streptokinase and produces a higher early coronary patency rate. Based on the favorable results of the Global Utilization of Streptokinase and Tissue Plasminogen Activator for Occluded Coronary Arteries (GUSTO) trial, t-PA is usually given in an accelerated regimen consisting of a 1- mg bolus, 50 mg iv over the initial 30 mins, and 35 mg over the next 60 mins; adjustment for weight is preferred for patients <67 kg. Allergic reactions do not occur because t-PA is not antigenic, but the rate of intracranial hemorrhage may be slightly higher than that with SK, around 0.7%.

Reteplase (r-PA), is a deletion mutant of t-PA with and extended half-life, and is given as two 10-mg boluses 30 mins apart. Reteplase was originally evaluated in angiographic trials which demonstrated improved coronary flow at 90 mins compared to t-PA, but subsequent trials showed similar 30-day mortality rates. Why enhanced patency with r-PA did not translate into lower mortality is uncertain.

Tenecteplase (TNK-tPA) is a genetically engineered t-PA mutant with amino acid substitutions that result in prolonged half-life, resistance to plaminogen-activator inhibitor-1, and increased fibrin specificity. TNK-tPA is given as a single bolus, adjusted for weight. A single bolus of TNK-tPA has been shown to produced coronary flow rates identical to those seen with accelerated t-PA, with equivalent 30-day mortality and bleeding rates. Based on these results, single-bolus TNK-tPA is an acceptable alternative to t-PA that can be given as a single bolus.

Other new thrombolytics include lanoteplase (n-PA), a deletion mutant of t-PA with prolonged half-life that is given as a single bolus (120,000 U/kg). Angiographic studies demonstrated increased TIMI 3 flow with n-PA compared to t-PA and an equivalent 30-day mortality rate, but a higher rate of bleeding. Staphylokinase, a plasminogen activator produced by certain strains of Staphylococcus aureus, is as potent as t-PA and significantly more fibrin-specific. Staphylokinase, however, has a short half-life, is antigenic, and induces antibody formation. Site-directed mutagenesis as well as conjugation with polyethylene glycol are being used in an attempt to reduce the immunogenicity of Staphylokinase and to increase its plasma half-life.

The ideal thrombolytic agent has not yet been developed. Newer recombinant agents with greater fibrin specificity, slower clearance from the circulation, and more resistance to plasma protease inhibitors are being studied.

## COMBINATION FIBRINOLYTIC AND ANTI-PLATELET THERAPY IN ACUTE ST-SEGMENT ELEVATION MYOCARDIAL INFARCTION

Thrombolytic monotherapy for acute ST segment elevation myocardial infarction is successful in achieving normal (TIMI grade 3) flow in only approximately 50%-60% of cases. Furthermore, fibrinolysis activates platelets, which causes further thrombus formation and subsequent reocclusion and reinfarction in a significant number of patients. Researchers have proposed that the combination of a glycoprotein IIb/IIIa inhibitor with a reduced dose of fibrinolytics would maximize inhibition of platelet aggregation without an increase in the most serious bleeding complications. Recent clinical trials have given some support to this hypothesis. In the Strategies for Patency Enhancement in the Emergency Department (SPEED) trial, TIMI 3 flow at 60 mins was achieved in 63% of patients at given half dose r-PA plus abciximab compared with only 48% of patients given full dose r-PA alone. Similarly, in the TIMI 14 Trial, flow was improved with the combination of abciximab and half-dose alteplase compared to full-dose alteplase alone at 60 and 90 mins, respectively. The GUSTO-IV-AMI is an international ongoing trial being conducted in 16,600 patients in 20 countries that will evaluate the use of half-dose reteplase and full-dose abciximab in acute ST segment elevation MI. "Facilitated" early percutaneous coronary intervention refers to planned percutaneous coronary intervention after reduced-dose pharmacological reperfusion therapy. Studies are currently underway to determine whether this combined approach could provide the optimal reperfusion strategy.

## PRIMARY ANGIOPLASTY IN ACUTE MYOCARDIAL INFARCTION

Rapid restoration of coronary blood flow is the initial goal of therapy for acute MI. As many as half to two thirds of patients presenting with acute MI may be ineligible for thrombolytic therapy, and these patients should be considered for primary PTCA. Primary PTCA can achieve reperfusion of the infarct vessel without the risk of bleeding associated with thrombolytic therapy. In experienced hands, initial success rates exceed 90%. Complications include reinfarction in 2% to 4% (a rate lower than with thrombolytics), distal embolization of thrombus, ventricular arrhythmias, and transient but severe hypotension associated with the Bezold-Jarisch reflex, which is more common with reperfusion of the right coronary artery.

The major advantages of primary PTCA over thrombolytic therapy include a higher rate of Thrombolysis in Myocardial Infarction (TIMI) trial grade 3 (normal) flow and a lower risk of intracranial hemorrhage. Several randomized trials have suggested that PTCA is preferable to thrombolytic therapy for AMI patients at higher risk, including those >75 yrs old, those with anterior infarctions, and those with hemodynamic instability. The largest of these trials is the GUSTO-IIb Angioplasty Substudy, which randomized 1,138 patients. At 30 days, there was a clinical benefit in the combined primary endpoints of death, nonfatal reinfarction, and nonfatal disabling stroke in the patients treated with PTCA compared to t-PA, but no difference in the "hard" endpoints of death and myocardial infarction at 30 days.

It should be noted that these trials were performed in institutions in which a team skilled in primary angioplasty for acute MI was immediately available, and that this allowed for prompt reperfusion of the infarct-related artery. More important than the method of revascularization is the time to revascularization, and this should be achieved in the most efficient and expeditious manner possible. If primary PTCA can be performed in a timely manner (within 60 mins) by highly experienced personnel, this may be the preferred method of revascularization, since it offers more complete revascularization with improved restoration of normal coronary blood flow and detailed information about coronary anatomy. When performing PTCA will require a substantial time delay, and in less experienced hands, thrombolytic therapy may be preferable. Retrospective studies have suggested that in the community setting (as opposed to PTCA performed as part of a controlled clinical trial), mortality rates after MI with routine primary PTCA and thrombolytic therapy are currently equivalent.

### Situations in Which PTCA Is Clearly Preferable to Thrombolytics in Acute Myocardial Infarction

- Contraindications to thrombolytic therapy
- Cardiogenic shock
- Patients in whom uncertain diagnosis prompted cardiac catheterization which revealed coronary occlusion

### Situations in Which PTCA May Be Preferable to Thrombolytics in Acute Myocardial Infarction

- Elderly patients (>75 yrs)
- Hemodynamic instability
- Large anterior infarction
- Patients with a prior MI or prior coronary artery bypass grafting

## SHCORONARY STENTSING FOR ACUTE MYOCARDIAL INFARCTION

Primary angioplasty for acute MI results in a significant reduction in mortality but is limited by abrupt vessel closure, recurrent in-hospital ischemia (10%-15% of patients), reocclusion of the infarct related artery (10%-15%), and restenosis in 30% to 45% of patients during routine angiographic follow up at 6 months. The PAMI Stent Trial was designed to test the hypothesis that routine implantation of the an intracoronary stent would reduce angiographic restenosis and improve clinical outcomes compared to primary balloon angioplasty alone. This large, randomized, multicenter trial involving 900 patients did not show a difference in mortality at 6 months, but did show improvement in ischemia-driven target vessel revascularization and less angina in the stented patients compared to PTCA alone.

Glycoprotein IIb/IIIa receptor antagonists inhibit the final common pathway of platelet aggregation, and their use in percutaneous intervention is becoming almost routine. The ReoPro and Primary PTCA Organization Randomized (RAPPORT) Trial compared the glycoprotein IIb/IIIa inhibitor abciximab to placebo in 483 patients with acute ST-segment elevation MI undergoing primary PTCA. The trial showed no difference in the primary endpoint of death, nonfatal MI, or any repeat revascularization procedure at 6 months, but the incidence of death, reinfarction, or urgent revascularization was lower with abciximab vs. placebo at 7 days; bleeding complications, which occurred mostly at arterial access sites, were more common with abciximab. The ADMIRAL Trial (Abciximab Before Direct Angioplasty and Stenting in MI Regarding Acute and Long Term Follow Up) is the first placebo controlled study to evaluate abciximab as an adjunct to primary PTCA and stenting in acute MI patients. Preliminary results showed that abciximab used in conjunction with stenting resulted in a nearly 50% relative risk reduction in the incidence of death, recurrent MI, and urgent revascularization at 30 days, although this was associated with an increased incidence of minor bleeding.

Complete results of this and other trials should help clarify the role of IIb/IIIa inhibition and primary stenting in acute MI.

## OTHER INDICATIONS FOR ANGIOPLASTY IN ACUTE MYOCARDIAL INFARCTION

In patients who fail thrombolytic therapy, salvage PTCA is indicated, although the initial success rate is lower than that of primary angioplasty, reocclusion is more common, and mortality is higher. The RESCUE trial focused on a subset of acute MI patients with anterior infarction and showed a reduction in the combined endpoint of death or congestive heart failure at 30 days in the group receiving salvage PTCA. There is no convincing evidence to support empirical delayed PTCA in patients without evidence of recurrent or provokable ischemia after thrombolytic therapy. The TIMI IIB trial and others studies suggest that a strategy of "watchful waiting" allows for identification of patients who will benefit from revascularization.

## MEDICAL THERAPY FOR MYOCARDIAL INFARCTION

### Aspirin

In patients who fail thrombolytic therapy, salvage PTCA is indicated, although the initial success rate is lower than that of primary angioplasty, reocclusion is more common, and mortality is higher. The RESCUE trial focused on a subset of acute MI patients with anterior infarction and showed a reduction in the combined endpoint of death or congestive heart failure at 30 days in the group receiving salvage PTCA. There is no convincing evidence to support empirical delayed PTCA in patients without evidence of recurrent or provokable ischemia after thrombolytic therapy. The TIMI IIB trial and others studies suggest that a strategy of "watchful waiting" allows for identification of patients who will benefit from revascularization.

# MEDICAL THERAPY FOR MYOCARDIAL INFARCTION

## Aspirin

Unless contraindicated, all patients with suspected MI should be given aspirin, 160 to 325 mg. This should be accomplished within the first 10 mins of hospital evaluation and the aspirin should be chewed to accelerate absorption. Aspirin has been shown to reduce mortality in acute infarction to the same degree as thrombolytic therapy, and its effects are additive to thrombolytics. In addition, aspirin reduces the risk of reinfarction.

Once begun, aspirin should probably be continued indefinitely. Aspirin irreversibly inactivates platelet cyclooxygenase, inhibiting platelet aggregation and reducing the release of platelet-derived vasoconstrictors such as serotonin and thromboxane A2. Recent data suggest that the anti-inflammatory effects of aspirin may play a role in inhibiting plaque rupture as well. Toxicity with aspirin is mostly gastrointestinal; enteric-coated preparations may minimize these side-effects.

## Heparin

Administration of full-dose heparin after thrombolytic therapy with t-PA is essential to diminish reocclusion after successful reperfusion. Dosing should be adjusted to weight, with a bolus of 80 U/kg and an initial infusion rate of 18 U/kg/hr, with adjustment to keep the partial thromboplastin time (PTT) between 50 and 70 secs. Heparin should be continued for 24 to 48 hrs.

Low-molecular-weight heparins (LMWH) have several theoretical advantages over unfractionated heparin. Because of a higher resistance to inactivation by platelet factor 4 and a lower affinity for heparin-binding proteins, LMWHs have a more predictable pharmacokinetic profile, greater bioavailibility, and longer plasma half-life, all of which result in more predictable and reliable anticoagulant effects.

LMWHs may be given once or twice daily as subcutaneous injections at fixed or weight-adjusted doses, thus simplifying administration and eliminating the need for laboratory monitoring and dose adjustment.

LMWHs have been studied in several large randomized trials in patients with unstable angina or non-Q wave MI. In both the Efficacy and Safety of Subcutaneous Enoxaparin in Non-Q-Wave Coronary Events (ESSENCE) study and the TIMI 11B trial, the combined endpoint of death, MI, or recurrent ischemia at 14 days was significantly reduced (15% relative risk reduction) with enoxaparin therapy compared to unfractionated heparin. The data regarding other LMWHs have not been as positive as the enoxaparin data, with no significant benefit from dalteparin treatment in patients already on aspirin. There are specific considerations with the use of LMWH, including decreased clearance in renal insufficiency and the lack of a commercially available test to measure its anticoagulant effect.

## Nitrates

Nitrates have a number of beneficial effects in acute MI. They reduce myocardial oxygen demand by decreasing preload and afterload, and may also improve myocardial oxygen supply by increasing subendocardial perfusion and collateral blood flow to the ischemic region. Occasional patients with ST elevation due to occlusive coronary artery spasm may have dramatic resolution of ischemia with nitrates. In addition to their hemodynamic effects, nitrates also reduce platelet aggregation. Despite these benefits, the recently reported GISSI-3 and ISIS-4 trials failed to show a significant reduction in mortality from routine acute and chronic nitrate therapy. Nonetheless, nitrates are still first-line agents for the symptomatic relief of angina pectoris and when MI is complicated by congestive heart failure.

Our practice is to administer sublingual nitroglycerin to all patients presenting with chest pain, unless the systolic blood pressure is <100 mm Hg or evidence of right ventricular infarction is present. For patients with persistent chest pain, intravenous nitroglycerin is infused at 10 &g/min and increased in increments of 5 to 10 &g/min every 5 mins until the pain resolves.

The major adverse effects of nitrates are hypotension and headache. Nitrates should be used with great caution in patients with right ventricular infarction, who may not tolerate decreases in filling pressure. Similarly, precipitous decreases in blood pressure in patients presenting with inferior MI should raise the suspicion of right ventricular involvement. Nitrate-induced hypotension is usually caused by vasodilation and is treated with rapid bolus infusion of intravenous fluids.

## Blockers

The blockers are beneficial both in the early management of myocardial infarction and as long-term therapy. In the pre-thrombolytic era, early intravenous atenolol was shown to significantly reduce reinfarction, cardiac arrest, cardiac rupture, and death. For patients receiving t-PA, immediate -blockade with metoprolol resulted in a significant reduction in recurrent ischemia and reinfarction.

Administration of intravenous -blockade should be strongly considered for patients presenting with acute myocardial infarction, especially those with continued ischemic discomfort and sympathetic hyperactivity manifested by hypertension or tachycardia. Therapy should be avoided in patients with moderate or severe heart failure, hypotension, severe bradycardia or heart block, and severe bronchospastic disease. Metoprolol can be given as a 5-mg iv bolus, repeated every 5 minutes for a total of 3 doses. Because of its brief half-life, esmolol may be advantageous in situations were precise control or the heart rate is necessary or rapid drug withdrawal may be needed if adverse effects occur.

Oral -blockade should be initiated in all patients who can tolerate it, even if they have not been treated with intravenous -blockers. The major side effects include exacerbation of heart failure, hypotension, conduction abnormalities, and bronchospasm.

## Angiotensin-Converting Enzyme Inhibitors

Angiotensin-converting enzyme (ACE) inhibitors are known to reduce mortality and improve symptoms in patients with symptomatic left ventricular dysfunction from a variety of causes, and to prevent progression to symptomatic heart failure in patients with asymptomatic left ventricular dysfunction. Several large randomized trials, most recently the Heart Outcomes Prevention Evaluation (HOPE ) study, have demonstrated that ACE inhibitors decrease mortality after MI. This improved survival is additive to the benefits of aspirin and -blockers. The mechanisms responsible probably include limitation in the progressive left ventricular dysfunction and enlargement (remodeling) that often occur after infarction, but a reduction in ischemic events was seen as well. Recent studies have suggested that ACE inhibition can ameliorate endothelial dysfunction in atherosclerosis.

Although the trials have demonstrated a benefit with ACE inhibition for all patients postinfarction, patients with significant left ventricular dysfunction (ejection fraction <40%) have the most to gain. ACE inhibition should be started early, preferably within the first 24 hrs after infarction. Immediate intravenous ACE inhibition with enalaprilat has not been shown to be beneficial. Patients should be started on low doses of oral agents (captopril 6.25 mg three times daily) and rapidly increased to the range demonstrated beneficial in clinical trials (captopril 50 mg three times daily, enalapril 10 to 20 mg twice daily, lisinopril 10 to 20 mg once daily, or ramipril 10 mg once daily).

## Calcium Antagonists

Randomized clinical trials have not demonstrated a mortality benefit for calcium-channel blockers for routine use after myocardial infarction. In fact, meta-analyses suggest that high doses of the short-acting dihydropyridine nifedipine increase mortality in MI. Adverse effects of calcium-channel blockers include bradycardia, atrioventricular block, and exacerbation of heart failure. Patients with non-Q-wave MI who are not in congestive heart failure, however, appear to have a significant reduction in reinfarction and recurrent ischemia when treated with diltiazem.

Although routine administration of calcium blockers in acute MI is not indicated, these agents are useful for patients whose postinfarction course is complicated by recurrent angina, because these agents not only reduce myocardial oxygen demand but inhibit coronary vasoconstriction. For hemodynamically stable patients, diltiazem can be given, starting at 60 to 90 mg orally every 6 to 8 hrs. In patients with severe left ventricular dysfunction, long-acting dihydropyridines without prominent negative inotropic effects such as amlodipine, nicardipine, or the long-acting preparation of nifedipine may be preferable; increased mortality with these agents has not been demonstrated.

## Antiarrhythmic Agents

Routine prophylactic administration of lidocaine is no longer recommended. Even though lidocaine increases the frequency of premature ventricular contractions and of early ventricular fibrillation, overall mortality is not decreased. In fact, meta-analyses of pooled data have demonstrated increased mortality from the routine use of lidocaine.

Nonetheless, lidocaine infusion is clearly indicated after an episode of sustained ventricular tachycardia or ventricular fibrillation, and should be considered in patients with nonsustained ventricular tachycardia. Lidocaine is administered as a bolus of 1 mg/kg (not to exceed 100 mg), followed by a second bolus of 0.5 mg/kg 10 minutes later, along with an infusion at 1 to 3 mg/min. Lidocaine is metabolized by the liver, and so lower doses should be given in the presence of liver disease, in the elderly, and in patients who have congestive heart failure severe enough to compromise hepatic perfusion. Toxic manifestations primarily involve the central nervous system, and can include confusion, lethargy, slurred speech, and seizures.Because the risk of malignant ventricular arrhythmias decreases after 24 hrs, lidocaine is usually discontinued after this point. For prolonged infusions, monitoring of lidocaine levels (therapeutic between 1.5 and 5 g/mL) is sometimes useful.

Intravenous amiodarone is an alternative to lidocaine for ventricular arrhythmias. Amiodarone is given as a 150 mg iv bolus over 10 mins, followed by 1 mg/min for 6 hrs, then 0.5 mg/min for 18 hrs.

Perhaps the most important point in the prevention and management of arrhythmias after acute MI is maintaining normal serum potassium and magnesium levels. Serum electrolytes should be followed closely, particularly after diuretic therapy. Routine administration of magnesium has not been shown to reduce mortality after acute MI, but empiric administration of 2 g of iv magnesium in patients with early ventricular ectopy is probably a good idea.

## COMPLICATIONS OF ACUTE MYOCARDIAL INFARCTION

### Postinfarction Angina and Infarct Extension

Causes of ischemia after infarction include decreased myocardial oxygen supply due to coronary reocclusion or spasm, mechanical problems which increase myocardial oxygen demand, and extracardiac factors such as hypertension, anemia, hypotension, or hypermetabolic states. Nonischemic causes of chest pain, such as postinfarction pericarditis and acute pulmonary embolism, should also be considered.

Immediate management includes aspirin, -blockade, iv nitroglycerin, heparin, consideration of calcium-channel blockers, and diagnostic coronary angiography.

Postinfarction angina is an indication for revascularization. PTCA can be performed if the culprit lesion is suitable, recognizing that acute outcomes and long-term patency may not be as good as those with elective angioplasty. CABG should be considered for patients with left main disease, three-vessel disease, and those unsuitable for PTCA. If the angina cannot be controlled medically or is accompanied by hemodynamic instability, an intra-aortic balloon pump should be inserted.

### Ventricular Free Wall Rupture

Ventricular free wall rupture typically occurs during the first week after infarction. The classic patient is elderly, female, and hypertensive. Free wall rupture presents as a catastrophic event with shock and electromechanical dissociation. Salvage is possible with prompt recognition, pericardiocentesis, and thoracotomy. Emergent echocardiography or pulmonary artery catheterization can help make the diagnosis.

### Ventricular Septal Rupture

Septal rupture presents as severe heart failure or cardiogenic shock, with a pansystolic murmur and parasternal thrill. The hallmark finding is a left-to-right intracardiac shunt ("step-up" in oxygen saturation from right atrium to right ventricle). It can be difficult to distinguish from mitral regurgitation on pulmonary artery catheter tracing. Both can produce dramatic "v" waves in the pulmonary artery occlusion pressure (PAOP) tracing. Echocardiography can help make the distinction. Surgical repair is required.

### Acute Mitral Regurgitation

Papillary muscle dysfunction is common after inferior MI but is rarely important hemodynamically; the characteristic holosystolic apical murmur of mitral regurgitation is typically present. Papillary muscle rupture, on the other hand, presents dramatically with marked hemodynamic compensation; consisting of pulmonary edema and shock; a murmur may or may not be present due to decreased cardiac output. Acute management includes afterload reduction with nitroprusside and intra-aortic balloon pumping as temporizing measures. Definitive therapy is surgical valve repair or replacement.

### Right Ventricular Infarction

Right ventricular infarction occurs in as many as 30% of patients with inferior infarction and is clinically significant in 10%. Patients present with hypotension, elevated neck veins, and clear lung fields. Although these patients appear to be in cardiogenic shock, right ventricular infarction carries a better prognosis.

The diagnosis is made by identifying ST elevation in right precordial leads or by characteristic hemodynamic findings on right heart catheterization (elevated right atrial and right ventricular end-diastolic pressures with normal to low PAOP and low cardiac output). Echocardiography can demonstrate depressed right ventricular contractility and can help differentiate right ventricular infarction from tamponade, which may present with similar clinical and hemodynamic findings.

Treatment, in addition to rapid reperfusion of the occluded coronary artery if necessary, includes fluid resuscitation with normal saline boluses to increase left ventricular filling pressure and inotropic therapy with dobutamine or possibly amrinone to stimulate RV contractility. Patients who do not respond rapidly to fluids need hemodynamic monitoring to guide therapy. For continued hemodynamic instability, intra-aortic balloon pumping may be useful, particularly because elevated right ventricular pressures and volumes increase wall stress and oxygen consumption and decrease right coronary perfusion pressure, exacerbating right ventricular ischemia. Nitrates should be avoided because of their propensity to reduce right ventricular preload, resulting in decreased cardiac output.

## Cardiogenic Shock

Cardiogenic shock as a complication of acute MI carries a high mortality rate, approaching 60% to 90% in some series. It is considered in detail on acute heart failure in the intensive care unit. Hemodynamically, cardiogenic shock is defined as a cardiac index <1.8 L/min/m2 with an elevated PAOP, generally >18 mm Hg. Prompt reperfusion of the occluded coronary artery is the only way to reduce the mortality associated with cardiogenic shock. Because thrombolytic therapy alone does not appear to be very effective in cardiogenic shock, primary PTCA is recommended. An intra-aortic balloon pump should be placed before the PTCA to stabilize the patient and enhance coronary blood flow and reduce myocardial oxygen demand. Urgent coronary artery bypass surgery may be an alternative if prompt angioplasty is not feasible.

## KEY POINTS

- Myocardial infarction is diagnosed by a compatible clinical history, evolution of characteristic ECG changes, and an increase and decrease in cardiac enzymes.
- All patients with suspected myocardial ischemia should be given aspirin upon presentation to the emergency department.
- Acute reperfusion of the occluded coronary artery is the key to achieving a good outcome. The promptness of reperfusion is more important that the mode by which it is accomplished.
- Thrombolytic therapy should be considered up to 12 hrs after the onset of symptoms.

- All patients should receive -blockers after acute myocardial infarction, except those who cannot tolerate them.
- Routine prophylactic administration of lidocaine is no longer recommended. Keep the serum potassium levels high. Consider administration of magnesium in patients with frequent ventricular ectopy.
- Patients with cardiogenic shock should be stabilized with an intra-aortic balloon pump and revascularized if possible by angioplasty or bypass surgery.
- Echocardiography is extremely useful for the diagnosis of complications after myocardial infarction. Invasive hemodynamic monitoring may be necessary in some cases as well.
- Prognosis after myocardial infarction is most closely related to the degree of left ventricular impairment.
- Not all akinetic myocardium is dead after myocardial infarction; consider the presence of myocardial stunning or hibernation.

## Chapter 8

# Sedation and Analgesia in Intensive Care

## INTRODUCTION

Pain and agitation are common in critically ill patients. The stress response causes tremendous neurohumoral elevations of plasma catecholamine, cortisol, glucose, antidiuretic hormone, and acute phase protein levels. These elevations can result in tachycardia, hypertension, vasoconstriction, increased oxygen consumption, salt and water retention, and blunting of the immune response. The primary goals of sedation and analgesia are to relieve pain and anxiety, attenuate the stress response, and improve compliance with care. In certain situations, neuromuscular blocking agents are necessary. Appropriate use of these medications requires a thorough understanding of drug indications, metabolism, side effects, and monitoring techniques.

## SEDATION

The Joint Commission on Accreditation of Health Care Organizations has defined four levels of sedation: minimal, moderate, deep, and general anesthesia (table 1). Sedated patients should be drowsy but arousable and able to follow commands. In certain patients, especially those who are asynchronous with controlled modes of mechanical ventilation ("fighting the ventilator") or in whom decreased oxygen consumption is desired, a deeper level of sedation is required. In general, sedation should be accompanied by analgesia because analgesics potentiate the effect of sedatives, resulting in lower sedative dose requirements.

**Table 1.** Levels of sedation.

| |
|---|
| ***Minimal sedation (Anxiolysis)*:**<br>Patient responds normally to verbal commands. Cognitive function may be impaired, but ventilatory and cardiovascular functions are unaffected.<br>***Moderate sedation or analgesia (Conscious Sedation)*:**<br>Patient responds purposefully to verbal commands with or without light tactile stimulation. Spontaneous ventilation is adequate, and cardiovascular function is maintained.<br>***Deep sedation or analgesia:***<br>Patient is not easily aroused but responds purposefully to painful stimulation. Patient may not be able to maintain a patent airway, and spontaneous ventilation may be inadequate. Cardiovascular function usually is maintained.<br>***Anesthesia*:**<br>Consists of general anesthesia and spinal or major regional anesthesia. It does not include local anesthesia. Patients are not arousable, even by painful stimulation. The patient often requires assistance in maintaining a patent airway and positive pressure ventilation. Cardiovascular function may be impaired. |
| *Adapted from Joint Commission on Accreditation of Health Care Organizations. Standards and intents of sedation and anesthesia. Comprehensive accreditation manual for hospitals: the official handbook. Chicago: The Joint Commission, Jan 1, 2001 Update.* |

Sedation needs vary over the course of a patient's stay in an intensive care unit (ICU). In the acute phase, a profound stress response may require deeper sedation and higher doses of analgesics. When a plateau is reached, sedative and analgesic requirements may decrease, but delirium may emerge. In the recovery phase, sedation and analgesia are tapered and discontinued.

In 1995, a Society of Critical Care Medicine (SCCM) task force (1) recommended midazolam hydrochloride (Versed) and propofol (Diprivan) for short-term sedation, lorazepam (Ativan) for longer-term sedation, and haloperidol (Haldol) for delirium. Most ICUs do not follow these recommendations, and sedative and analgesic regimens vary widely. Dasta and colleagues (2) reported the use of up to 23 different drugs in one surgical ICU. Lack of a standardized approach to sedation and analgesia can lead to polypharmacy, overmedication or undermedication, and increased cost.

Several scales have been used to assess the adequacy of sedation in ICUs. The most common observational scales are either graded or additive; caretakers rate the degree of sedation according to the patient's response to stimuli. With graded (single-category) scales, the degree of sedation is ranked along a graduated scale. The simple-to-use Ramsay scale (table 2) is the most common graded scale; the desired score depends on the indication for sedation. With additive (multiple-category) scales, the level of sedation is ranked by the sum of scores in several categories. The increased numbers of categories with additive scales improve validity but make this type of scale too cumbersome for routine use.

**Table** 2. Modified Ramsay scale for rating sedation

| *Indication* | *Score* |
|---|---|
| Anxious, agitated, restless | 1 |
| Awake, cooperative, oriented, tranquil | 2 |
| Semi asleep but responds to commands | 3 |
| Asleep but responds briskly to Glabellar tap or loud or loud auditory stimulus | 4 |
| Asleep with sluggish or decreased response to glabellar tap or loud auditory stimulus. | 5 |
| No response can be elicited | 6 |

Observational sedation scales are useless in patients receiving neuromuscular blocking agents. Blood pressure and heart rate are objective indicators but may be affected by underlying illness and drugs. Crippen (3) pioneered the use of continuous neurologic monitoring with processed electroencephalography, particularly during neuromuscular blockade. Bispectral processed electroencephalographic monitoring has been correlated with observational sedation scales and is especially useful in deeply sedated or paralyzed patients (4).

## Benzodiazepines

The benzodiazepines, which have anxiolytic and amnestic properties and anticonvulsant effects, are commonly used for sedation in ICUs. They undergo hepatic metabolism, some to active metabolites that may accumulate in the presence of renal and hepatic insufficiency. The most reliable and effective route of administration is intravenous, because the absorption of oral and intramuscular doses may vary. Benzodiazepines may be given intravenously by either intermittent bolus dosing or continuous infusion. Disadvantages of intermittent boluses include the need for high nursing input and the risk of underdosage or overdosage.

With continuous infusions, bolus doses are given to obtain the desired level of sedation, and infusion is used to maintain that level. The continuing need for infusion as well as the dose should be reassessed daily; the infusion rate is decreased when sedative requirements are stable over a 24-hour period (5). Daily interruption of infusions, when feasible, may decrease the duration of mechanical ventilation and the length of ICU stay (6). Tolerance occurs with prolonged administration, and withdrawal syndrome may accompany rapid discontinuation of the drug.

Three benzodiazepines—diazepam (Valium), lorazepam, and midazolam—are available for parenteral use.(table 3). Onset and duration of action are determined by lipid solubility. Respiratory depression and hypotension are dose-dependent. Hypotension occurs primarily in hypovolemic patients and is potentiated by the concomitant use of opioids.

**Table 3.** Comparison of parenteral benzodiazepines.

| *Drug* | *Onset (min)* | *Half-life (hr)* | *Equivalent dose (mg/kg IV)* | *Average bolus dose (mg IV)* | *Comments* |
|---|---|---|---|---|---|
| Diazepam (Valium) | 3-5 | 20-66* | 0.3-0.5 | 2-20N | ot recommended for continuous infusion |
| Lorazepam (Ativan) | 10-20 | 10-20 | 0.05 | 1-4 | Drug of choice in hepatic failure; may accumulate in renal failure |
| Midazolam HCl (Versed) | ≤3 | 1-4 | 0.15-0.3 | 1-5 | Peripheral distribution prolongs effects; may accumulate in hepatic and renal failure |

**Upper value is average of maximum half-lives of drug and its active metabolite, desmethyldiazepam.*

## Diazepam

Diazepam has an onset of action of 3 to 5 minutes and a half-life of 20 to 36 hours. This water-insoluble drug is metabolized by the liver to an active metabolite, desmethyldiazepam, which has a half-life of 48 to 96 hours. Diazepam is not recommended for continuous infusion.

## Midazolam

Midazolam has a rapid onset and short elimination half-life. It is water-soluble and can be administered intravenously without irritation. It is metabolized by the liver to the less potent 1-hydroxy-midazolam. Accumulation can occur in the setting of renal and hepatic failure. Midazolam is the most potent amnestic and produces greater decreases in blood pressure in hypovolemia than does diazepam. Despite the relatively short half-life of midazolam, extensive distribution can cause prolonged sedation. Recovery time is proportional to the infusion's duration; therefore, midazolam infusion generally should not exceed 48 hours.

### Lorazepam

Lorazepam, a highly lipophilic benzodiazepine, is a more potent amnestic than diazepam. Lorazepam is metabolized by the liver to inactive metabolites. The half-life of lorazepam is prolonged in the setting of renal failure. Nevertheless, lorazepam is the benzodiazepine of choice in liver failure. Lorazepam is the preferred benzodiazepine for long-term sedation (>48 hours) (1). It is water-insoluble and is dissolved in a propylene glycol carrier. Propylene glycol toxicity is possible with high-dose infusions.

### Benzodiazepine Reversal

Flumazenil (Romazicon) is a competitive antagonist of benzodiazepine effects. It is administered intravenously at a dose of 0.2 mg and increased to a maximum of 1 mg, which may be repeated at 20-minute intervals to a maximum dose of 3 mg/hr. Its duration of antagonism is short. With longer-acting benzodiazepines, resedation may result. Caution is needed with long-term benzodiazepine use, because withdrawal seizures may occur.

## OTHER SEDATIVES

Barbiturates and ketamine hydrochloride (Ketalar) are no longer commonly used for sedation in ICUs. Etomidate (Amidate), a short-acting sedative used for rapid-sequence intubation, can produce adrenocortical suppression after a single dose, making it inappropriate for use in critically ill patients (7).

### Propofol

Propofol (2,6-di-isopropylphenol) was introduced in 1989 as an anesthetic induction agent. It has a rapid onset of action and short half-life. Propofol has amnestic effects, but not to the degree of benzodiazepines. It is metabolized at least partially by the liver to inactive metabolites and excreted by the kidneys; however, the presence of renal or hepatic dysfunction does not significantly affect clearance. Propofol can accumulate in peripheral tissues, prolonging sedative effects. Tolerance to the drug has been reported after more than 7 days of use but may occur sooner.

Adverse effects include hemodynamic and respiratory depression, pain with peripheral administration, and green discoloration of the urine. Hypotension, a common side effect, is dose- and rate-dependent. Propofol is dissolved in a lipid emulsion, and prolonged infusion (>72 hours) requires frequent monitoring of triglyceride levels to avoid pancreatitis. This risk may be reduced by using the 2% rather than the 1% formulation (8). Microbial contamination of the lipid emulsion is a significant risk, and the infusion setup must be changed every 12 hours.

The SCCM task force has recommended propofol or midazolam for short-term sedation (<48 hours). Several studies have found that propofol and midazolam provide equally effective sedation. With propofol the time to extubation is shorter once the drug is discontinued, but the degree of hypotension and cost are higher than with midazolam. The cost may be offset by a longer ICU stay with midazolam, especially when used for longer than 48 hours; however, supporting data are insufficient.

### Haloperidol

Haloperidol is a butyrophenone derivative with a half-life of 14 hours. It is used for the treatment of delirium (not associated with alcohol withdrawal) in ICUs. Although not approved by the US Food and Drug Administration for intravenous administration, it has been shown in many studies to be safe when administered by this route.

Hypotension may occur in hypovolemic patients. QT-interval prolongation, torsades de pointes, and neuroleptic malignant syndrome are infrequent but life-threatening adverse effects. The recommended dose for intermittent intravenous administration is 1 to 10 mg every 4 to 12 hours.

## ANALGESIA

Patients in ICUs may experience pain related to underlying illness or injury, medical procedures, and therapies, causing anxiety and discomfort, interference with sleep, prevention of early mobilization, and augmentation of the stress response. In patients with multiple organ system derangements, treatment of pain may compromise other system functions (causing, for example, respiratory depression or hypotension), and agents must be chosen with this in mind.

Opioid analgesics are the drugs of choice for pain relief in the critically ill. The mu and kappa opioid receptors mediate narcotic analgesic effects. Binding of the mu receptor by agonists such as morphine sulfate causes analgesia, respiratory depression, and euphoria. Opioid analgesics are metabolized primarily by the liver and excreted in the urine. Tolerance may develop with prolonged administration.

Routes of administration vary, but narcotic analgesics are most commonly given intravenously, by either intermittent bolus or continuous infusion. The intravenous route is preferred in ICU patients because absorption may vary with other routes. In alert patients, continuous patient-controlled analgesia can be accomplished by intravenous or epidural administration. Patient-controlled analgesia allows adjustment of narcotic medication within preset limits, decreases nursing burden, and reduces patient anxiety over inadequate or untimely delivery of analgesics.

The intrathecal or epidural route can be used for administration of narcotics or local anesthetics. This mode is most effective in postoperative patients; it should be avoided in critically ill patients who are immunocompromised or who have coagulopathy, because epidural hematoma or abscess may result. Anesthetics can cause early respiratory depression, and narcotics can cause late respiratory depression.

A stable blood level can be maintained by delivery of a constant infusion of drug that matches the rate of metabolism. Unfortunately, there is no way to presumptively determine the ideal rate of administration in individual patients. Pain threshold and rate of metabolism or drug excretion can vary among patients and in a single patient as a result of organ system dysfunction and development of tolerance to the drug. Ideal administration of analgesics entails rapid adjustment to the desired effect, maintenance of that level with minimal intervention, and rapid dissipation of the effect once the drug is discontinued. The use of intermittent intravenous boluses requires constant vigilance and thus is labor-intensive; in addition, a constant level of analgesia is difficult to achieve. It is important that continuous infusion be preceded by bolus dosing to achieve the desired level of analgesia; a constant level can then be maintained with continuous infusion.

Monitoring of analgesia in the critically ill is difficult. Reliable, objective measures of pain are unavailable, and underlying disease or medications may alter blood pressure and heart rate, which are commonly used indicators in noncommunicative patients. The visual analogue scale is a useful tool for assessing pain in patients who are awake and communicative, which is often not the case in ICUs.

## Side Effects

The major dose-limiting side effect of opioid analgesics is respiratory depression. Some narcotics, especially morphine and meperidine (Demerol) hydrochloride, may cause histamine release, resulting in pruritus, hypotension, and smooth muscle contraction. Opioids blunt the cough reflex and the sensation of dyspnea, an effect that can be advantageous, especially in mechanically ventilated patients.

All narcotics, particularly the phenyl piperidines, can cause muscle rigidity, which may interfere with respiration. Hypotension generally occurs only in hypovolemic patients or in patients receiving very large intravenous doses. Narcotics reduce gastrointestinal motility and may cause nausea, vomiting, or ileus. Smooth muscle contraction may result in contraction of the bladder sphincter and urinary retention.

Systemic side effects are minimized with epidural or intrathecal administration. Common side effects associated with these delivery modes include pruritus, nausea and vomiting, respiratory depression, and urinary retention (which occurs in up to 80% of patients).

### Morphine and Meperidine

Morphine is the narcotic analgesic of choice in ICUs. It has a rather slow onset owing to its lipid solubility. A potent metabolite, morphine-6-glucuronide, can accumulate in the setting of renal failure and cause prolonged sedation. The active metabolite of meperidine, normeperidine, can accumulate and cause tremor, pupillary dilatation, and seizures. Doses should be reduced in patients with renal insufficiency.

### Phenyl Piperidines

The phenyl piperidines, which are mu-receptor agonists, include fentanyl (Sublimaze), alfentanil hydrochloride (Alfenta), and sufentanil citrate (Sufenta). Phenyl piperidines are more potent than morphine and have a faster onset of action. Fentanyl is the opioid analgesic of choice in patients with hemodynamic instability (1). Despite the drug's short half-life, redistribution into peripheral tissues occurs and can cause prolonged effects. Fentanyl has an active metabolite that may accumulate in renal failure. Alfentanil has no active metabolite, making it the drug of choice in renal failure. All phenyl piperidines are considerably more expensive than morphine.

## Narcotic Reversal

Naloxone hydrochloride (Narcan), an opioid-receptor antagonist, reverses most of the effects of narcotics. Intravenous doses of 0.4 to 2.0 mg are used. Smaller doses can reverse respiratory depression without affecting analgesia. Depending on the half-life of the analgesic used, naloxone may require additional dosing.

## Nonnarcotic Agents

Nonsteroidal anti-inflammatory drugs (NSAIDs) are mild analgesics that inhibit prostaglandin synthesis. Prostaglandins appear to be involved in the smooth muscle contraction seen in renal and biliary colic, conditions in which these agents are particularly effective. In addition to having anti-inflammatory activity, NSAIDs are antipyretic and inhibit platelet aggregation; they do not cause the sedation, respiratory depression, and hypotension that are common with opioid analgesics. Major side effects are platelet dysfunction, renal dysfunction, and gastrointestinal ulceration or irritation. NSAIDs are limited by the lack of intravenous formulations; however, ketorolac tromethamine (Toradol) may be administered intramuscularly or intravenously. In some patients, regionally injected local anesthetic blocks can reduce or eliminate the need for narcotic analgesics, control postoperative pain, attenuate the neurohumoral response to stress, and provide analgesia and anesthesia for invasive procedures.

# NEUROMUSCULAR BLOCKADE

Appropriate sedation and analgesia methods are usually adequate to control agitation in patients in an ICU. However, neuromuscular blockade is necessary in certain situations:

- Severe acute respiratory distress syndrome requiring inverse-ratio ventilation or permissive hypercapnia
- Severe respiratory failure requiring improved chest wall compliance

- Facilitation of independent lung ventilation
- "Inappropriate" reflex hyperventilation (central nervous system disease)
- Excessive shivering
- Need for immobility (for magnetic resonance imaging, computed tomographic scanning, tracheostomy)
- Tetanus or neuroleptic malignant syndrome

Neuromuscular blocking agents interfere with the action of acetylcholine on postsynaptic receptors at the neuromuscular junction. The agents are either depolarizing or nondepolarizing; the latter are used in ICUs. Neuromuscular blocking agents should be added only when sedation and analgesia have failed; they should never be used without concurrent sedation and analgesia.

Neuromuscular blocking agents may be used to reduce oxygen consumption; control intracranial pressure; or facilitate endotracheal intubation, unconventional modes of mechanical ventilation, or procedures that require complete immobility. These agents can facilitate mechanical ventilation by inducing patient-ventilator synchrony, but attempts must be made to ascertain and correct the reason the patient is in asynchrony. Recognition of the serious side effects of neuromuscular blocking agents has led to more conservative use of these drugs in recent years.

Previously, bolus dosing was preferred to continuous infusion because of the risk of overparalysis. However, the availability of relatively inexpensive peripheral nerve stimulators for monitoring the degree of neuromuscular blockade has facilitated the use of continuous infusion. Infusions should be stopped once every 24 to 48 hours, when possible, to reassess the continuing need for paralysis. Frequent suctioning, prophylaxis for deep venous thrombosis, and vigilant monitoring for inadvertent disconnection from mechanical ventilation are essential. In addition, care should be taken to prevent pressure ulcers and peripheral nerve damage.

## Prolonged Weakness in Neuromuscular Blockade

At least two mechanisms explain long-lasting weakness after neuromuscular blockade. The first is prolonged drug action in patients with difficulty clearing the drug, such as those with renal or hepatic insufficiency, for hours to days after discontinuation. Some patients may experience effects for months. The second is use of corticosteroids, particularly those given in high doses for more than 24 to 48 hours. These drugs appear to act synergistically with neuromuscular blocking agents to cause a severe form of myopathy. Affected patients exhibit an acute myopathy characterized by elevations in serum creatine kinase levels and muscle fiber atrophy and necrosis. Serum creatine kinase levels should be monitored in all patients receiving neuromuscular blocking agents plus corticosteroids. Risk factors for persistent neuromuscular blockade include renal and hepatic dysfunction, concomitant use of aminoglycoside antibiotics or high-dose corticosteroids, and metabolic acidosis.

## Depolarizing Neuromuscular Blocking Agents

These agents bind the postsynaptic acetylcholine receptor and transiently and irreversibly depolarize the neuromuscular junction; they are degraded by plasma cholinesterase. Succinylcholine chloride (Anectine, Quelicin) is the only available depolarizing neuromuscular blocking agent. With a quick onset and short duration of action, succinylcholine is commonly used for rapid-sequence intubation; however, serum potassium concentration can increase by 0.5 to 1.0 mEq/L. Because of the risk of hyperkalemia, succinylcholine should not be used in patients with renal failure or with increased numbers of acetylcholine receptors (eg, patients with spinal cord injury, neuromuscular disease, trauma, burns [more than 5 days after injury]). Succinylcholine should not be used for continuous infusion in ICUs.

## Nondepolarizing Neuromuscular Blocking Agents

These agents antagonize the action of acetylcholine at the neuromuscular junction. Hemodynamic effects and duration of action vary among neuromuscular blocking agents (table 4); the drugs are classified as short-, intermediate-, or long-acting. Short-acting agents, such as rocuronium bromide (Zemuron) and mivacurium chloride (Mivacron), have an onset of action similar to that of succinylcholine. However, short duration of action and high cost make these drugs impractical for continuous infusion in ICUs.

**Table 4.** Comparison of commonly used nondepolarizing neuromuscular blocking agents

| *Drug* | *Onset (min)* | *Duration (min)* | *Loding dose (mg/kg)* | *Infusion rate* | *Metabolism excretion* | *Comparative cost* |
|---|---|---|---|---|---|---|
| Atracurium besylate (Tracrium) | 3-5 | 20-35 | 0.3-0.5 | 5-10H microg rams/ kg/min | offman elimination/ renal, biliary | $$$$ |
| Pancuronium bromide (Pavulon) | 3-5 | 60-90 | 0.04-0.1 | 0.06-0.1 mg/kg/ h | Hepatic/ rental | $ |
| Vecuronium bromide (Norcuron) | 3-5 | 20-35 | 0.06-0.1 | 1 micro grams/ kg/min | Hepatic/ biliary | $$$ |

Vecuronium bromide (Norcuron), atracurium besylate (Tracrium), and cisatracurium besylate (Nimbex) are commonly used intermediate-acting neuromuscular blocking agents. Vecuronium is effective in 3 to 5 minutes and has a duration of action of about 35 minutes. It has few cardiovascular side effects, except when combined with high-dose fentanyl or sufentanil infusion. Vecuronium may accumulate in the setting of renal or hepatic failure. Atracurium and cisatracurium are degraded by Hoffman elimination and ester hydrolysis and therefore do not exhibit half-life prolongation in patients with renal or hepatic failure. Laudanosine, a metabolite, may accumulate in renal failure and cause seizures; however, case reports suggest that clinical doses are unlikely to result in important central effects in humans (10). Cisatracurium is more potent than atracurium and does not cause the hypotension seen with high doses of that drug. Onset and duration of action are similar to those of vecuronium.

Pancuronium bromide (Pavulon), a long-acting medication, is by far the least expensive neuromuscular blocking agent used for continuous infusion in ICUs. It has a vagolytic effect on the sinus node and blocks the reuptake of norepinephrine. Tachycardia and hypertension are the major side effects. Resistance to paralytic effect may occur with prolonged use. Pipecuronium bromide (Arduan) and doxacurium chloride (Nuromax) are more potent and long-acting than pancuronium but are considerably more expensive.

## Monitoring of Neuromuscular Blocking Agents

When neuromuscular blocking agents are used, the degree of paralysis should be monitored with a peripheral nerve stimulator. The two most common sites for twitch monitoring are the ulnar nerve (adductor pollicis) and facial nerve (orbicularis oculi). Four electrical impulses are delivered over 2 seconds, a sequence known as *train of four*. In the absence of neuromuscular blockade, muscle contraction occurs with each stimulus (four twitches). The usual goal is to obtain one of four twitches, which corresponds to about 90% blockade.

If no twitches occur, the "tetanus mode" may be used. A 5-second stimulation generates a sustained twitch, after which the train of four sequence is repeated. If no twitches occur, the patient is overparalyzed and the neuromuscular blocking agent is discontinued until two of four twitches return. If one or two twitches occur on post-tetanic train of four, the agent is held or decreased until one or two twitches return on simple train of four.

With intermittent bolus injections, the train of four sequence should be performed every 30 to 60 minutes. No additional doses are given until one or two twitches reappear. If continuous infusion is used, the rate is adjusted to maintain the lowest dose that accomplishes the goal (usually one or two of four twitches). Compared with standard clinical dosing, train of four monitoring may result in the use of lower doses of neuromuscular blocking agents and faster recovery once the agents are discontinued, even in the presence of renal or hepatic failure (11). There is no evidence, however, that such monitoring reduces the risk of myopathy.

## SUMMARY

The stress response to critical illness can have many deleterious effects. Appropriate use of sedation and analgesia can attenuate the stress response, alleviate pain and anxiety, and improve compliance with care. Agitation responds best to anxiolytic drugs; pain is best relieved by analgesics. A combination of these drugs can act synergistically, because most analgesics provide some degree of sedation. In select cases, neuromuscular blocking agents are required, but they should not be used without concomitant sedation and analgesia. Use of agents needs to be tailored to the needs of individual patients; indications, anticipated length of need, and underlying organ system derangements are important considerations.

resources available for combatting death were so limited that physicians rarely faced painful choices about when to use them.

This medical acceptance of some illnesses as fatal occurred within a larger teleological worldview, within which death could be seen as a fitting and natural event that was not under human control. Death was regarded as a release from worldly troubles or as the first step in the transition to an afterlife. Comfort could be found in the idea of of death occurring within a planned universe, in which creatures lived and died according to their destinies. The notion of a "natural death" was an attempt to rob death of its sting by construing it as an event for which no one could be held responsible.

Remnants of this view can still be found in the distinction between natural and unnatural deaths—that is, those resulting from accidents or violence, in our contemporary medico-legal taxonomy. This terminology notwithstanding, however, modern medicine now assumes a less passive stance on death. Although medical technology has given the physician new power to sustain life, it is accompanied by the responsibility for deciding when it is to be used. Those who place the preservation of life above all other values contend that disease must always be treated aggressively. Increasingly, however, the imperative always to treat aggressively is coming to be viewed as indefensible. Critics condemn the needless, painful, and costly prolongation of the dying process for critically ill patients. The only advantage of this practice is that it provides a simple black-and-white response to a reality that contains many shades of grey, thus sparing physicians from having to make morally difficult choices. It is easy to sympathize with those who want to resist the slippery slope upon which determinations have to be made about the prolongation of life. However, few health care professionals working in intensive care environments believe that aggressive treatment is always morally appropriate.

# Chapter 9

# Death in the ICU

## INTRODUCTION

Death poses one of the most significant problems of human existence. Life is a precondition of virtually anything else a person might want; yet we know that death comes to us all eventually.

As biological events, disease and death are subject to control and manipulation by medical intervention. However, medicine can only hope to delay death, not eliminate it; time is on death's side in the long run. In fact, it is only in this century that the prolongation of life has become a primary goal of medicine, along with the relief of suffering. Previously, medicine could often promise little more than comfort. Before 1900, most people died from communicable diseases. The patient who received aggressive treatment was either restored to "good health" or not helped at all. Besides the minimization of suffering and disease, the Hippocratic writings mention the physician's duty to refrain from interfering with those who are succumbing to their diseases. Medicine held no hope for persons rendered critically ill by the breakdown of major body systems, and the medical

## DECISIONS ON DEATH IN INTENSIVE CARE SETTINGS

For patients receiving modern medical care, death is often not the result of inexorable processes that defy all treatment efforts; instead, death occurs because of human decisions to forego medical intervention at some point. According to the Commission for the Study of Ethical Problems in Medicine and Biomedical and Behavioral Research, "For almost any life-threatening condition, some intervention can now delay the moment of death." We can no longer derive comfort from the view that death is "natural.""Very little is 'natural' about our present day existence, and least natural of all is the prolonged period of dying that is suffered by so many incurable patients solicitously kept alive to be killed by their disease," writes Barrington. And Lasagna remarks, "In this age of surgical derring-do and widespread use of drugs, almost no disease can be said any longer to have a 'natural history.'"

Decisions to withhold life-prolonging therapies are sometimes construed as strictly factual judgments about a patient's unsalvageability." This is often an illusion, however. If a treatment can delay the moment of death, however slightly, then a responsible decision about whether to provide such treatment must be based on the assignment of values to the overall costs of the treatment and the possible benefits in terms of additional days or even hours of life.

In many cases, admission to an Intensive Care Unit (ICU) is the result of a preliminary decision about the appropriateness of aggressive treatment. Presumably, ICU care is intended to bring patients through crises to more stable conditions of health. However, since admission errors do occur and even carefully screened patients may get worse, physicians may have to consider withholding or withdrawing intensive efforts after the patient is in the ICU. It is somewhat ironic that such decisions, which are clearly moral and involve highly personal and individual values, are made by strangers who work in an environment that allows little time for reflection. Indeed, some decisions must be made after an emergency has arisen—for example, a cardiac arrest. Some have argued that physicians are trained to evaluate data and make decisions in such a way that value judgments are disguised as technical ones. In fact, a physician evaluating a situation from the clinical perspective may not even realize the significance of a decision, much less the contribution of values to the process. It is impossible, however, to make a nonarbitrary decision that is value-free.

## Patient Autonomy

While the physician's bias is (and should be) toward the preservation of life, the actual treatment decision is, in principle, the patient's responsibility. The principle of informed consent, which underlies treatment decisions, requires that after the competent patient has been provided with all relevant medical information, he or she has the right either to authorize or refuse any proposed treatment. Although the moral and legal right to forego life-sustaining treatment does theoretically belong to the competent patient, we will address a number of situations in which the implementation of this principle is anything but straightforward. Even when the competent patient makes a treatment decision, the physician bears the ultimate moral and legal responsibility for what is done. Nurses and other medical personnel are primarily responsive to the physician's orders, rather than to the patient's wishes. Moreover, it is the physician who must provide the patient with information, judge whether the patient is competent, and implement the patient's wishes. Thus, the principle of informed con sent notwithstanding, it is the physician who ultimately orchestrates the decisions and activities that determine the timing of the patient's death.

## Reasons for Withholding Life-Sustaining Therapies

Although there may be a number of factors influencing competent decisions to forego life-sustaining therapies, we will primarily be concerned with two general categories of reasons. A patient who still values life might opt to forego treatment because of its associated *burdens and benefits*—for example, invasiveness, painfulness, disfigurement, psychological costs, and expected gains in length and quality of life. The terminal cancer patient who is not eager to die but opts to forego radical chemotherapy treatments that might marginally prolong his or her life has made a decision on the basis of "burden of treatment" considerations. On the other hand, a patient who views his or her very existence as undesirable might opt to forego even a minimally burdensome treatment—as an example, a patient who declines antibiotic treatment in the event of an infection. Such a patient is avoiding the burden of further life, not the burden of treatment. Such factors will hereafter be referred to as "burden of life" considerations.

The underlying principle we will argue for here is simple—that is, a rational decision to undertake life-sustaining therapies should depend only upon whether the patient stands to benefit from the therapies. The central issue is whether, given the patient's values, the potential benefits outweigh the burdens associated with the therapy. Although most of us agree in general about what is burdensome and what is beneficial, these assessments may differ in particular cases. Differences may be due to such factors as willingness and ability to tolerate pain, reasons for living, or different religious views or beliefs about death. For example, a Jehovah's Witness may decide that the burden of receiving blood products outweighs the benefits of surviving a medical crisis and prolonging life significantly. Adhering to the principle of informed consent optimizes the possibility of using the patient's own values as a guide for treatment.

Of course, abundant uncertainty surrounds any medical decision. Unless the patient is faced with an immediately life-threatening condition, it is impossible to predict the future precisely. Specifically, neither the effectiveness nor the burdensomeness of possible interventions is completely predictable. In the ICU setting, these problems are intensified. Patients may have to consider foregoing expensive, traumatic, and perhaps fatal treatment that offers only the hope of salvaging an already compromised life condition.

**Two Kinds of Complications**

Any number of factors may operate to complicate the ICU physician's attempt to respect patient autonomy regarding potential lifeprolonging therapies. These factors can be divided into two categories: those having to do with the physician's determination of the patient's competence to make such a decision, and those having to do with influences that may affect the competent patient. We will consider each of these in turn.

*Assessment of Patient Competence*

A person who is critically ill is unlikely to display the characteristics usually associated with cool rationality. His pain, anxiety, depression, and/or sedation may lead the physician to question the patient's competence to make any important treatment decisions on his own behalf. Further, technical factors such as intubation or extreme weakness may prevent even a competent person from being able to communicate clearly. For these reasons, the physician has the ultimate moral and legal responsibility for determining that the decision to forego life-prolonging treatment represents the considered choice of a competent individual.

Detailed examination of problems associated with the assessment of competence is beyond the scope of this work. In general, the problem of assessing competence becomes critical only when there is some divergence of opinion about a particular treatment; if physician, family, and patient all agree on the desirability of a particular treatment, it is unlikely that the issue of competence will even be raised. Where no consensus is reached, a psychiatric consult can be helpful and is certainly prudent. Should an incompetent patient refuse treatment that is clearly appropriate, a court order may be sought.

One way of dealing with the general problem of competence in critically ill patients is for persons to specify their treatment wishes before reaching a stage of terminal or critical incapacity. The living will is a document that can be used to communicate such decisions to the family, physician, lawyer, or clergy. In some states, "right to die" legislation has been passed which gives living wills legal force. Even this approach is not free of problems, however, for it is impossible to anticipate the specifics of a medical crisis. The physician must still determine whether the patient has reached the condition he had in mind when he specified his wishes.

### *Influences on the Competent Patient*

Even if the patient is alert, understands his situation, and can communicate his wishes clearly, the physician must still give careful attention to the views and role of family members. They naturally have a strong interest in the patient's situation, and are apt to influence his decision in a time of crisis. The physician may suspect that the patient's expressed wish is the result of family coercion, as well as concern for family members. He must also realize that complying with a patient's decision to forego treatment may provoke legal action by angry and resentful relatives, who may later claim that the patient's treatment refusal did not reflect a competent decision.

Family members are not the only ones whose values may influence the patient's decision. Because the physician occupies a position of special responsibility, authority, and privilege, he usually has the greatest influence on patient and family decisions. If the physician is not sensitive to the need to respect patient autonomy, his own values will probably determine the course of treatment. The patient's decision about whether to authorize treatment must be based primarily on information provided by the physician. As a matter of practical necessity, physicians will always fall short of the theoretical ideal of fully informing the patient, and their choices about what information to provide may be biased in favor of treatment.

In some cases, the patient does not volunteer opinions, nor is he questioned, on these matters. Family members who are only aware that the patient is critically ill urge the physician to "do everything he can" to pull the patient through the crisis. As long as there is a reasonable chance that the patient may recover, it may seem unnecessary to raise questions with the family or patient about abandoning aggressive treatment.

A combination of these factors frequently accounts for the physician's being the first to consider the possibility of withholding therapy. Often the physician's bias in favor of doing everything possible for the patient prevails until it appears that recovery is very unlikely. At this point, both the substance and the tone of communications with the patient and family change and the orchestration of death begins. The physician and other caregivers begin to prepare everyone involved for the realization that available therapies no longer promise significant improvement. Differing perceptions and attitudes among family members must be addressed and, if possible, resolved. A psychiatrist may be helpful at this point in determining what the patient has understood and where he stands. The social worker may help the patient and family to understand and accept the bleaker prognosis, and arrive at a consensus on what option to pursue. Nurses, of course, play central roles in every stage of these delicate tasks of informing, assessing comprehension, and hearing the patient's decision.

## THE MORAL DECISION

Thus far we have been focusing primarily on the setting in which decisions to forego life-prolonging therapies take place, and the different roles, values, and expectations which the various participants may bring to such decisions. We have tried to emphasize both the importance of patient autonomy and the fact that respect for this autonomy does not override the physician's ultimate responsibility for both making and implementing the decision to forego life-prolonging therapy, which leads to the patient's death. We must now examine some of the reasons behind decisions to terminate treatment.

We argued above that responsible decisions to terminate treatment are similar to most other decisions in that they ultimately involve a burden/benefit analysis. We normally place such a high value on human life that it seems repugnant to speak of assigning a value to its prolongation. Unless one is to pursue aggressive treatment in every case without regard for any of its associated burdens, the prolongation of life must be evaluated. If such an assignment of value is not shared by the patient, this strategy violates individual autonomy.

There are two results of burden/benefit analysis which would warrant the withholding of life-sustaining treatments: the burden of treatment might be so great as to outweigh the benefit of prolonging life; or, life itself might be seen as a burden which would be magnified by even a minimally burdensome life-prolonging treatment.

A variety of factors conspire to cloud thinking and inhibit rational decision making in these contexts. The patient or family may be plagued by guilt and denial, which may preclude their acknowledging responsibility for making the decision. Those involved may welcome any misconstrual of the situation that disguises the magnitude of the decision that has to be made. As a result, a number of considerations often creep into the decision making process that tend to be irrelevant, are sometimes obfuscatory, and are usually counterproductive to a rational outcome. These considerations are expressed as various dis tinctions—that is, between "ordinary" and "extraordinary" means or therapies; the intended consequences of a therapy and those which are merely foreseen; withdrawing a life-prolonging therapy which has already been initiated and withholding such a therapy in the first place; actively killing a critically ill patient and passively allowing such a patient to die. While none of these distinctions speaks in any straightforward way to the burdens or benefits of life-prolonging therapies, each is sometimes held to be morally significant. We will examine each of these distinctions in turn.

## THERAPIES

The decision to withhold life-sustaining treatment is sometimes based on the claim that the treatment at issue would constitute "heroic" or "extraordinary" means. There are two completely different interpretations of those terms in this context. "Extraordinary" sometimes means "very unusual." Some treatments are, therefore, extraordinary in that they are highly unusual, exotic, or still experimental. Alternatively, a treatment may be extraordinary in that it is exceptionally burdensome in the broadest sense—that is, very painful or unpleasant, risky, expensive, demanding of time and/or labor, or otherwise difficult to provide.

The setting in which medical care is being provided may, of course, determine what is extraordinary in either of these senses. In the ICU of a teaching hospital, the use of exceedingly complex and costly equipment is routine; in a bush hospital, use of an IV catheter might be extraordinary in both senses. No procedure is inherently extraordinary; this will always depend upon the context.

Can the mere fact that a life-prolonging treatment is extraordinary in either of these senses ever provide sufficient justification for withholding it. Surely the fact that the procedure is unusual, highly exotic, or still experimental could not do so by itself. The appropriateness of any treatment, routine or otherwise, depends only on whether its benefits outweigh its burdens in the particular situation. It would be inappropriate to withhold a potentially beneficial therapy merely because it was unusual.

Historically, the emphasis has been primarily, but not exclusively, on the second interpretation of extraordinary—that is, burdensome. McCartney provides an excellent historical discussion of this distinction. It was introduced in the late sixteenth century, when the Catholic church first indicated that the prolongation of life by means of extraordinarily burdensome surgical procedures (those which were extraordinarily risky, painful, or disfiguring) was not morally obligatory. Pope Pius XII's 1957 pronouncement also indicated there was no obligation to prolong life if it required treatments that were extraordinarily burdensome.

But how burdensome is "too burdensome." We have already seen that it is appropriate to withhold a treatment only if the burden it imposes outweighs its benefits. If calling a treatment "extraordinary" only means "more burdensome than beneficial in this particular case," then the fact that it is extraordinary is not what justifies its being withheld; in this context, the use of the term "extraordinary" adds nothing to the analysis that cannot be said more clearly by speaking directly of burdens and benefits. In fact, there seem to be two dangers in using the term "extraordinary" to refer to a treatment as probably being more burdensome than beneficial in some particular situation. The first is that it may mislead people into thinking that the treatment should be withheld simply because it is so exotic. The second is that it tends to obscure the extent to which a treatment must be burdensome before it ought to be withheld. The fact that it is extraordinarily burdensome only justifies its being withheld if the treatment does not also promise an extraordinary benefit. The burdens of amputation, toxic chemotherapy, or dialysis are obviously very great. But such therapies are often appropriate precisely because they also provide great benefits. Thus, at best, referring to such treatment as "extraordinary" adds nothing to what can be said more precisely by speaking of burdens and benefits; at worst, it suggests either that a treatment may be withheld simply because it is exotic, or that a treatment may be withheld simply because it is very burdensome. Since neither of these facts alone constitutes a good reason for withholding any therapy, we suggest that use of the term "extraordinary" is counterproductive. Optimal medical diagnosis requires the honest acknowledgment of even those medical facts which are unpleasant and the avoidance of irrelevancies. Similarly, optimal moral reasoning about the value of preserving a life requires that the relevant value judgments be faced squarely, and not obscured in ways that invite confusion of moral and technical judgments.

## CONSEQUENCES

It is sometimes proposed that it is not permissible to withhold a life-sustaining treatment (or administer a potentially lethal dose of a narcotic) if the patient's death is intended; such actions may be permissible if the death is merely a foreseeable consequence of what is intended—that is, the relief or minimization of suffering. This distinction is also suspect, however. It is true that our moral evaluations of harmful actions sometimes depend upon an agent's intentions, and certainly our evaluations of agents depend upon them. We are inclined, for instance, to tolerate the unintended harmful effects of insecticides on crops if their use is necessary to maximize the crop yield, but would certainly condemn anyone who introduced poisons into the environment simply for the purpose of causing harm. (Similarly, we would probably condemn a sadistic dentist who intentionally and gleefully inflicted pain in the course of doing excellent dental work, even if he inflicted no more pain than any other dentist.)

Some people, however, have mistakenly inferred that a person is responsible only for what he directly intends, so long as the intended good consequences of his action outweigh the foreseen, but unintended, harm. Thus, a physician who intends to keep a suffering patient free from pain is not held morally responsible if the patient dies because a burdensome treatment was withheld, or because an analgesic caused respiratory depression. In fact, this argument is sometimes used to show that such a physician has not killed his patient. It is, of course, absurd to suggest that people can only be said to have done what they *did intentionally*. If this were the case, drunken drivers could not be said to cause car accidents, and persons who engage in irresponsible sex could not be considered accountable for the unintended pregnancies that sometimes result.

We suggest that this use of the distinction between what is intended and what is foreseen is not legitimate. First, it is often impossible to distinguish between the foreseen and intended consequences of an action. For example, does the abortionist who crushes the fetus' skull *intend* its death, or merely foresee it as an undesirable consequence of reducing the size of its head. Second and more important, agents are generally responsible for all of the reasonably foreseeable consequences of their actions, even if they clearly do not intend them. Acknowledgment of this principle is implied by our expectation that an agent will weigh all of the costs associated with some action which he or she believes will achieve some good. The person who spends family funds wisely is still responsible for the diminution of the account balance.

This does not mean that all actions having harmful consequences are blameworthy. A harmful action may be acceptable if its performance will fulfill an obligation, or if the harm is seen as a worthwhile means of achieving a benefit. This point is illustrated by the use of any burdensome therapy to benefit a consenting patient. Thus, although a dentist is responsible for the pain he inflicts, his actions are acceptable because the anticipated benefits outweigh the pain. (This conclusion assumes, of course, that the agent is not violating any duties in performing this action—for example, administering a potentially beneficial treatment to a competent patient without consent.)

The use of this distinction is particularly insidious because it typically serves only to obscure the proper focus of non treatment decisions—namely, whether the intended or merely foreseen burden of treatment is likely to outweigh the benefits. If this issue is not faced squarely, rational non treatment decisions will remain elusive.

## WITHHOLDING VERSUS WITHDRAWING

The distinction between withholding a life-sustaining therapy in the first place and withdrawing such a therapy once it has been initiated is widely believed to be morally significant. Many medical personnel are quite comfortable with the idea of withholding a therapy to which a patient has not given consent, but are reluctant to withdraw a life-sustaining therapy that is already in place—even if the patient decides that he or she wants it withdrawn. We wish to argue that this, too, is a mistake. Since the factors underlying the intuitive belief in the moral significance of this distinction are somewhat subtler and more complex than those in the first two cases, our criticisms must be correspondingly more elaborate. We offer three criticisms:

The first criticism is that the distinction itself is vague, and cannot always be made with certainty. Never starting a patient on a ventilator, renal dialysis, or antibiotics constitutes withholding treatment; removing a patient from a ventilator exemplifies withdrawing treatment. But what if a series of individual treatments (for example, renal dialysis, injections of insulin, antibiotics) is discontinued, or a pacemaker battery or IV drip is not replaced. In answer to these questions, it has been suggested that if some action is required, lack of compliance could be construed as "withdrawing"; if no action is required, one is "withholding" treatment. It is certainly true that one may psychologically *feel* more responsibility for doing something that requires physical action. Nevertheless, this explanation cannot bear the moral weight ascribed to it by those who endorse this distinction. Otherwise, the many cases involving patients on ventilators (which physicians are reluctant to disconnect even though life on the ventilator has become unacceptably burdensome for the patient) could easily be resolved by replacing their power switches with 24-hour "timer" switches, which would require daily resetting in order to continue treatment. Since treatment would be stopped without any physical action, not resetting the machine could be construed as withholding treatment. But surely it is absurd to suggest the resolution of any moral problem through "technological" means. Physicians who refrained from resetting such "timer" switches would surely be just as responsible for the lack of ventilator function as those who turn off more conventional ventilators. Although consideration of this hypothetical solution shows that the presence or absence of physical action does not make the moral difference, it is difficult to understand how the distinction between "withholding" and "withdrawing" can be understood more precisely.

The second criticism is that physicians are generally willing to withhold or withdraw therapies that they believe are not or will not be beneficial; it is not clear why the case should be different with nonbeneficial *life-sustaining* therapies. The initiation or continuation of *any* treatment should depend upon whether its potential benefits outweigh its associated burdens, a principle which is violated by the continuation of some life-sustaining therapies. One possible rationale for exempting life-sustaining therapies from this criterion of usefulness is that if they are withdrawn the patient will die. However, death is often an acceptable—perhaps even desirable—consequence of withholding treatment. Why, then, should it become so problematic in the case of treatment withdrawal. If the treatment is clearly nonbeneficial and merely prolongs a burdensome life, the fact that the person will die without it should become a reason *for*, not *against* its withdrawal. The physician who persists in such a treatment clearly violates the injunction to do no harm, regardless of whether the treatment is lifesustaining.

The third criticism is that other patients may be harmed by the physician's attachment of moral significance to the distinction between withholding and withdrawing treatment. Sometimes an uncertain, but potentially life-saving, treatment (for example, use of a ventilator) which might get a patient past a crisis is not undertaken because the physician believes that the therapy will have to be continued as long as it is sustaining the patient's life—even if the underlying condition does not improve. The perceived risk of ending up with a patient who is ventilator-dependent, will never recover, and who will find life on a ventilator burdensome may prompt the decision to withhold the potentially life-saving treatment in the first place. Sometimes physicians make this determination. In other cases, patients refuse a potentially life-saving therapy rather than risk the possibility of spending the final weeks of their life on a ventilator. It is difficult to imagine a stronger criticism of any alleged "moral principle" than to show that its implementation sometimes foreseeably leads patients to refuse potentially beneficial treatments.

Given these criticisms, one might ask why anyone would think the distinction between withholding and withdrawing treatment had a moral significance in the first place. It might be because of the psychological association with "action" vs. "inaction." Soldiers commonly believe that it is less psychologically traumatic to destroy entire villages from an altitude of 30,000 feet by pressing a button, than to have to kill one enemy woman or child face-to-face. We have already seen, however, that the distinction between withholding and withdrawing therapy cannot be clearly defined in terms of the presence or absence of any physical action.

Another possible explanation is that this intuitive belief derives from a failure to distinguish between the physician's two different levels of commitment. When a physician takes on a case, he or she becomes committed to offering the patient continued medical care, and incurs an obligation not to abandon the patient. In another sense, by initiating a *course* of treatment, rather than a single attempt, a physician becomes committed to the entire effort. The former "commitment" is clearly moral—that is, one incurs an ongoing moral obligation to provide the patient with needed medical care. The latter, however, is something quite different. By "committing oneself" to a course of treatment, the physician assumes the moral obligation to persevere with the treatment even if it has proven to be ineffective or counterproductive. By their very nature, some projects require sustained effort if they are to succeed (for example, losing weight, saving money, completing college, treating an infection with antibiotics). By and large, it is this fact that is being acknowledged when people speak of "being committed to a course of action." Simply making a commitment neither precludes the possibility nor absolves one from the responsibility of abandoning a project at any stage. Only extraordinarily perverse logic could lead someone to conclude that a physician's commitment to a patient entailed a commitment to continue a course of treatment that was clearly harmful.

More generally, anyone who embarks upon any course of action behaves irrationally if he or she perseveres after it becomes clear that the course of action has become counterproductive. A person who does so when acting as another person's agent is behaving both irrationally and immorally. This seems to be the case when a physician insists upon continuing life-sustaining therapy when it is no longer in the patient's best interest.

Finally, it might be suggested that the intuition gains its force from the fact that the withdrawal of life-prolonging therapy seems to involve killing the patient, while withholding only involves letting the patient die; killing someone is morally worse than merely letting someone die. Let us examine the role of this latter distinction in termination-of-treatment decisions.

## KILLING VERSUS LETTING DIE

The common intuition that there is an important distinction between killing and letting die seems to apply whether the death at issue is bad, as most deaths are, or good, as death would be for a patient whose life had become a burden. Intuitively, it seems that it is virtually never right to kill someone except in self-defense. However, most people will readily agree that, under certain circumstances, it may be morally permissible to let someone die—for example, in cases of the sort we have been discussing or when someone cannot be rescued without great danger to the potential rescuers. Although most physicians would never consider administering poison in order to kill a terminally ill patient, they would readily consider refraining from resuscitation attempts if there was no hope of substantial recovery. Thus, it seems that killing and letting die can not be morally equivalent. We must consider two serious criticisms of this deep-rooted intuition.

While the terms "killing" and "letting die" are *sometimes* used in a purely descriptive way, that is often not the case, especially in medical contexts. When they are not used descriptively, they can obscure moral assumptions. Let us first consider situations in which the terms are being used descriptively. In general, if someone performs an action which causes a person's death, we say that he killed the person; if someone refrains from acting to prevent a death, we say that he allowed the person to die. Thus, for instance, an assailant killed his victim when he shot him, but a patient who refused to be put on a ventilator was allowed to die of respiratory failure.

When critically ill patients die, however, it is frequently difficult to know which of these characterizations is a more accurate description. In these cases, a death may be characterized as "killing" or "letting die" only *after* it has been assessed morally; while the term that is used will simply *reflect* that evaluation, it will simultaneously appear to *justify* it. The moral assessment is apt to be more dependent upon the particular responsibilities of the persons involved than on whether they "performed an action" or "refrained from acting." If, for instance, a physician on duty in an emergency room stood by idly while an accident victim bled to death, we would consider him blameworthy and might even go so far as to say that his negligence killed the patient. Consider a patient who dies because the ventilator is withdrawn. If a hired assassin crept into the hospital and decided to bring about the intended death of his victim by disconnecting the ventilator, we would certainly say that the assassin had killed the patient and was guilty of homicide. If, on the other hand, a physician had removed the ventilator at the request of his competent patient, we would say that the patient's death had been allowed, though not caused, by the physician. Which is it when "surgical misadventure" results in a patient's death. If we suspected the surgeon of greed and carelessness, we might well say that he had killed the patient; if we view the situation as an unavoidable accident for which the surgeon could not have been expected to prepare, we may simply say that the patient died from complications of his disease. In these cases, then, the choice between "killing" and "letting die" is not merely a matter of description; it involves a normative element. The normative force of these two terms conveys the moral evaluation that has already been reached about the death.

Naturally, this evaluative use of one of these terms is more likely to occur in cases that are ambiguous or unclear from the beginning. But many cases that involve the withholding or withdrawing of lifeprolonging therapy are also ambiguous. Indeed, our tendency to use these terms to reflect our prior moral assessments of particular cases is so great that even the administration of lethal doses of narcotics is seldom interpreted as an example of a physician killing a patient; rather, such cases are routinely interpreted in ways that obscure the fact that the patient has been killed. In summary, then, we must be wary of attempts to condemn or justify particular treatment/nontreatment options on the grounds that the proposed course of action would either amount to killing or merely letting the patient die. This terminology is more apt to conceal than to elucidate the real basis for the moral judgment that is being made.

The second criticism of the killing/letting die distinction acknowledges the possibility of there being a distinction, but denies that it has any intrinsic moral significance. This criticism has been advanced by a number of philosophers, most prominently in an important article by James Rachels.

Rachels claims that incidental features of various cases mislead us into believing there is an inherent moral difference between killing and letting die. In most actual cases of killing, the agent acts from malevolent motives and does serious harm to his victim. Rachels suggests it is these common, but logically incidental, features of most killings that make them morally wrong. When we hear of cases in which someone is allowed to die, on the other hand, these features are usually not present. We are most apt to hear about benevolent caregivers who attempt to help a suffering patient by refraining from action that would only prolong his or her misery.

Rachels asks us to consider various pairs of cases in which these incidental differences are minimized, to see whether our intuitive reaction changes. For example, he uses two cases which include the features that make most killing wrong. The first case involves a greedy uncle who drowns his nephew in the bath in order to gain an inheritance. In the second case, the uncle approaches the child in the bathtub with the intention of drowning him. When he discovers, to his delight, that the boy has slipped in the tub and is drowning accidentally, he stands by until the child is dead. Surely, argues Rachels, the two cases contain equal amounts of moral evil; the uncle's action in the first is no worse than his inaction in the second. He also offers two cases which lack these morally objectionable features. In the first case, a terminally ill patient's caregivers allow him to die slowly by withholding treatment for pneumonia. The caregivers in the second case administer a lethal injection to a similarly suffering patient in order to put him out of his misery. The motive in each case is to minimize the patient's suffering. But this motive is served even better in the second case, where the patient is actively relieved of the burden of a painful life in such a way that his total suffering is reduced even further. Rachels believes that in this case killing may actually be preferable to allowing someone to die. Since this seems perfectly obvious in the case of suffering animals, why should it be so hard to grasp in the case of humans suffering terminal illness. The simple answer, "We value life," cannot be correct, for that consideration would apply equally against killing and letting die.

Finally, Rachels points out that what amounts to inaction under some circumstances may constitute action under other conditions. Rachels notes that the AMA opposes "the intentional termination of the life of one human being by another." He argues, however, that physicians are simply deluding themselves if they believe that by respecting the killing/letting die distinction they absolve themselves of the charge of intentional termination of life. Just as We may intentionally insult a person by refusing to shake his hand, a physician may intentionally terminate a suffering patient's life by withholding a lifeprolonging therapy. Consider, for instance, an advanced and miserable Alzheimer's patient who has contracted an infection; a decision not to administer antibiotics amounts to a decision to terminate the patient's life intentionally. Since the desirability of the patient's death is the motivating factor in the decision, treatment is withheld in *order that* the patient will die sooner than he would if treated.

How sound is Rachels' criticism of the primitive intuition that killing is intrinsically worse than letting die. Rachels' arguments certainly do suggest that part of the reason we view killing as worse is based on features of the situations that are accidental to the killing/ letting die distinction. But has Rachels shown that, in the context of critically ill patients, the distinction is never of any moral significance. We must tease apart a number of subtle issues that are intertwined here. First, it must be noted that Rachels has *not* shown that in *all* situations in which it would be right to let a patient die, it would also be right to kill that patient. At most, this will be so only when the reason for letting the patient die is that life itself has become a burden. In cases where treatment is withheld because the *treatment* is too burdensome—for instance, the cancer patient who would like to extend his or her life, but not at the expense of painful chemotherapy treatments, it would be absurd to suggest that since withholding treatment is justified, so is killing the patient. Thus, at best, Rachels' argument only holds in cases involving the patient's intended death. The cancer patient does not want or intend to die, even though he or she wants and intends to avoid the burden of painful chemotherapy. In light of this qualification, then, is his argument persuasive.

It is our view that neither the primitive intuition nor Rachels' view is completely correct. We suggest that both views are too simple in that both overlook the potential significance of special moral relationships among the persons involved. It is a mistake to think that the moral evaluation of actions or omissions that lead to a person's death depends only upon whether they are actions or omissions and the agent's motives. It is also essential to consider whether the parties have any special moral relationships which entail particular rights and duties.

Let us consider two cases involving parties with no special moral relationships. One person, through indifference, fails to aid another, whose life he could save at little or no cost to himself. His action is deplorable, but not as bad as that of a driver who indifferently kills a pedestrian he could have avoided hitting. Both cases involve the evil of a regrettable and easily avoidable death; the second involves the additional evil of interfering adversely in the welfare of another person in a way that violates that person's rights. Thus, when strangers are involved, the primitive intuition seems correct and Rachels is wrong; killing a stranger is worse than letting one die.

But physicians and their patients are engaged in a special moral relationship. The physician is the patient's agent and is responsible for his or her welfare. Here Rachels' argument may appear to have more substance, especially when death constitutes a harm to the patient. If any person who is responsible for another's welfare stands by while that person is harmed by influences such as disease that could easily be counteracted, such inaction is probably just a morally reprehensible as active killing.

Does the special moral relationship between physician and patient reinforce Rachels' argument that there is no difference between a physician's killing a patient and letting him or her die when the patient's death is a beneficial release from a burdensome life. Several philosophers believe that Rachels' claim rests on a misconstrual of the duties that form the basis of the doctor/patient relationship. Specifically, Bonnie Steinbock argues that Rachels is mistaken in stating that physicians withhold treatments and allow patients to die because they are motivated by either a duty or a benevolent impulse to see that the patient is relieved of a burdensome life. She claims that such a duty or impulse has no place in the ethics of the physician/patient relationship. Rather, physicians who withhold life-prolonging therapies are, or should be, motivated either by the desire to spare the patient the burden of painful treatment, or by a duty to respect the patient's right to refuse treatment. She argues that the right to informed consent gives the competent patient the right to refuse treatment, hence obliging the caregiver to withhold it; it does *not* give the patient the right to demand from his caregivers whatever might be to his benefit, including assistance in intentionally hastening his own death. Steinbock claims that physicians are not bound by any principles that require them to kill patients upon request. Such actions, she argues, would be totally contrary to the spirit of medicine, and should not be permitted under any circumstances.

In her critique of Rachels, Steinbock contends that physicians should never act or refrain from acting with the intention of hastening a patient's death. Her view is remarkable for two reasons. First, Steinbock has no quarrel with Rachels on one central point; she seems to accept Rachels' claim that there would be little moral distinction between what she calls passive and active euthanasia—that is, between a physician killing a patient while intending his or her death, and a physician withholding or withdrawing treatment while intending a patient's death. She grants that these might be morally equivalent, but then insists that *both* are wrong because they are incompatible with the moral principles that define the physician's role and the 1973 AMA code, which forbids "the intentional termination of the life of one human being by another."

Her argument with Rachels, then, focuses on whether physicians *ever* intend the deaths of their patients—regardless of whether treatment is withheld or withdrawn, or lethal doses of painkillers are administered. Her contention is that they do not. In order to maintain this view in the face of decisions by physicians to withhold antibiotics from advanced Alzheimer's patients, withdraw ventilators from patients in respiratory failure, and administer lethal doses of painkillers, Steinbock must rely very heavily on the "intended/foreseen" distinction.

The second remarkable feature of Steinbock's view, then, is her insistence that in each of these cases the death is merely foreseen and not intended. We noted earlier that this distinction this problematic. Although physicians may find it comforting to imagine that they never intentionally hasten the deaths of their patients, we doubt that this belief can often survive honest and critical scrutiny. Patients who refuse therapy or request painkillers in doses that may be lethal are often not the only ones who view their lives as burdensome; their families and physicians may share their belief that their deaths will be a desirable release from suffering. Under these circumstances, Steinbock's suggestion that such physicians do not intend the deaths which they are hastening seems ill-advised. An abortionist might similarly argue that he or she is not intentionally killing the fetus, but merely foresees its death as an inevitable consequence of suctioning it from the uterus. The political assassin might plausibly argue that he or she didn't intend to kill the president when he/she shot him, even though he or she did see his death as an inevitable consequence of removing him from office by putting a bullet through his heart. Also, one wonders what the physician in such cases does intend, if it is not the patient's death. According to Steinbock, the physician's intention is either to honor the patient's refusal of treatment, or to spare the patient the burden of the painful therapy that might prolong life. With the first possibility, Steinbock suggests that the physician, passive and duty-bound to honor the patient's wishes, stands back and lets the patient decide whether his or her life is to be prolonged. With the second possibility, Steinbock suggests that it is appropriate for the physician to be concerned with the minimization of suffering, and to participate in the burden-benefit analysis which determines whether the patient's life is worth prolonging, given the burden of treatment. It seems odd, however, to suggest that physicians participate in the process of assessing costs and benefits so selectively.

In all of this, Steinbock is driven to forced and implausible interpretations of decisions and intentions and their justifications. In order to insulate the physician from anything that can be construed as intending the patient's death, Steinbock recognizes, for instance, that in some cases *patients* may refuse treatment because they decide that they are better off dead. Given this fact, isn't it obvious that physicians may share this view with their patients-especially since they may well have a more accurate understanding than either the patient or the family of how bleak the patient's prognosis really is. And in such cases, isn't it undeniable that part of a physician's intention—for instance, in withholding an antibiotic from an advanced Alzheimer's patient—is to hasten the patient's death. This realization may be painful for the physician, for it forces him or her to acknowledge the taking of a particular stand on the straightforward moral dilemma concerning the conflicting imperatives to preserve life and minimize useless suffering. Once he or she has decided that the minimization of suffering has priority in a particular case, Rachels' central argument again becomes persuasive—that is, this goal can be realized even more quickly by killing the patient than by merely withholding life-prolonging therapy.

## THE FINAL ARGUMENT

This final argument on these issues is sometimes cited in defense of the prohibition on mercy killing, which Rachels is attacking. It also has application as part of a more comprehensive concern about termination-of-treatment decisions. The central premise is that the practice of medicine involves and requires a fundamental bias in favor of the preservation of life. Thus, even if Rachels is right about killing being the most compassionate and beneficial thing to do in certain individual cases, physicians should continue to respect the distinction (and, by parity of reasoning, the other distinctions we have criticized above), in order to prevent a general erosion of the respect for life which is essential to the practice of medicine. Steinbock alludes to, but does not develop, this argument in her critique of Rachels, and it recurs in one form or another throughout the literature. James Childress, for instance, writes, "Because the distinction between killing and letting die is inextricably tied up with our understanding of medical care, we cannot remove it without tearing the whole fabric. For the community or the medical profession to authorize physicians actively to kill patients would so alter the moral ethos of medicine as to necessitate a new basis of trust. Trust is the expectation that others will respect moral limits. . . . Trust in the context of medical care involves the expectation that medical practitioners will work for our health and life, will provide 'personal care,' and will do us no harm."

The claim that allowing mercy killing in some cases would lead to a general erosion of the respect for life is based on the belief that there is no clear way to distinguish between the cases in which mercy killing would be defensible and those in which it would not. According to the argument, we find a continuum of cases. Near the top of the "slippery slope," one finds the patient who is alert and clearly competent, terminally ill, and suffering intolerable and uncontrollable physical pain; because life has become burdensome, the patient wants to be released from his suffering. At the bottom of the "slope," there are helpless and dependent persons who may be incompetent, suffering nonterminal conditions that may involve only emotional distress, or who may even be fairly content, but whose continued existence inconveniences others. Rachels would presumably have physicians kill patients near the top of the slope; allowing such an action is a step onto a slope so slippery as to involve the risk of precipitating or "sliding into" the morally unacceptable killing of others further down the slope.

The slope is doubly slippery. First, the very terms used to describe the above continuum of acceptable to unacceptable killings are characterized by imprecision. How competent is "competent." How terminal is "terminal." While a patient in multiple system failure is obviously terminal, what of the newly diagnosed AIDS patient or the multiple sclerosis patient. How much pain is "intolerable." Considerable difficulties are encountered in defining competence and prognosis, with respect to both terminality and pain management; the determination of the quality of life of incompetent persons is even more difficult. Thus, even the most cautious and best-intended physician, who views all four of these conditions as necessary for actively killing a patient, will find these tests difficult to apply.

The other reason for the slope's being slippery is that each of these conditions can be challenged as being necessary for mercy killing. In fact, each of the four has been challenged by compassionate, wellintentioned thinkers. First, the condition of competence is not met by anencephalic neonates or comatose patients who have never voiced any opinions about the circumstances under which they would not want to be kept alive. If mercy killing can be beneficial to competent patients, why should it be denied as an option to proxies making decisions on behalf of similar patients who happen to be incompetent.

Secondly, although the condition of terminality is not met in any straightforward sense by persons with diabetes or emphysema, their right to refuse treatment guarantees their right to end their own lives intentionally. If we take this to be a right to mercy killing in the case of the terminally ill, why should we not extend it to patients who, although not yet near death, request suicide assistance.

Thirdly, the condition of *physical* pain seems arbitrary. It has been suggested that some persons who endure chronic emotional pain or anguish as the result of advanced dementia should be as eligible for mercy as those who have the good fortune to be suffering physically instead of mentally.

Fourth and last, while it may seem difficult at first to imagine that someone would justify mercy killing on the basis of a person's burdensomeness to others, this is often a reason for withdrawing ventilators from severely brain-damaged patients. It is difficult to construe such termination of treatment as beneficial to the patients, since it is doubtful whether the patients still embody a perspective from which anything could be either a benefit or a harm. While attention is given to any previously expressed wishes in such cases, it would be naive to suppose that none of the motivation for terminating treatment derived from concern for the family and others for whom scarce medical resources promise greater benefits.

Thus, each of these four conditions seems in some way relevant to distinguishing between morally justifiable and morally offensive killing. On closer scrutiny, however, it becomes clear that none provides a sure toehold for the well-intentioned physician who is lured onto the "slippery slope" by arguments such as Rachels', but who wants to guard against transforming medicine from a life-affirming institution into one in which there is not only little respect for life, but which freely dispenses death as well.

A natural extension of this argument applies to our previous criticisms of the other distinctions, since our attacks on each of them may be construed as contributions to the slipperiness of the slope. Physicians observing the distinction between ordinary and extraordinary therapies reflect medicine's life-respecting ethos by insisting upon treatment for patients suffering life-threatening conditions for which nonexotic treatments are available. Physicians relying heavily on the distinction between foreseen and intended consequences will reflect that ethos by administering lethal doses of morphine only to patients who are in serious pain. Physicians observing the distinction between withholding and withdrawing treatment will do so by refusing to withdraw life-prolonging therapy from those presently receiving it. Physicians who are persuaded by our arguments about the moral irrelevance of each of these distinctions for termination-of-treatment decisions will be much more inclined to opt for death than physicians who believe all of these distinctions are morally significant. Thus, according to the argument, in order to preserve the life-respecting ethos of medicine, physicians must continue to respect these distinctions and ignore as irrelevant (or perhaps denounce as subversive) the exhortations of medical ethicists to the contrary.

A final dimension of the slippery slope argument shifts the focus from the respect-for-life bias of medicine *as it guides physicians* to the *public perception* of that bias. According to this line of reasoning, public trust is obviously necessary if medicine is to be effective, since physicians generally treat only those persons who trust them enough to seek medical attention. But if the public begins to perceive physicians as dispensers of both death and life, this confidence in medicine will be eroded and health care will obviously suffer as a result. Childress construes patient trust in medical practitioners as the belief that they will "work for our health and life." David Louisell develops this theme: "Euthanasia would threaten the patient-physician relationship: confidence might give way to suspicion . . . Can the physician, historical battler for life, become an affirmative agent of death without jeopardizing the trust of his dependents." Patients who already view hospitals as places where people die, *in spite* of what can be done, will come to realize they are also places where people are sometimes killed intentionally. The cost of this shift in perception in terms of the public trust is thus an additional consideration against liberalizing physicians' views and termination-of-treatment decisions.

Two fundamental strategies have been adopted by theorists responding to this slope argument. The bolder of the two embraces a position which the proponents of the argument see as unacceptably far "down the slope." Mary Rose Barrington acknowledges that her argument for mercy killing entails a radical revision in the way we think about death. She grants, for instance, that her vision includes the possibility of people viewing doctors as dispensers of death. She insists, however, that such a possibility, far from eroding trust, would provide comfort and reassurance to anyone concerned about possibly being subjected involuntarily to the pain and indignity of a protracted death in an intensive care setting. (There is no evidence that the hospice movement has tarnished public trust in medicine, in spite of the fact that its underlying ethos renounces the goals of restoring health and prolonging life, and substitutes the more modest and attainable goals of comfort and "supportive care.") Barrington even accepts the possibility that those who are both elderly and infirm might some day feel obligated to step aside voluntarily and gracefully, rather than insisting upon the use of every possible intervention to eke out a few more days of life, however marginal, at costs, however staggering-especially in the face of competing demands for limited medical resources. Barrington would presumably see this as indicative of a need for the infirm and critically ill to speculate about whether it was their duty to step aside, instead of clinging to life until every conceivable resource for its prolongation has proven futile.

A different response to the slope argument is offered by Daniel Maguire. He also grants the slipperiness of the slope, but argues that morality in an open society depends upon learning to negotiate slippery slopes responsibly, rather than simply avoiding them. Maguire dismisses the view that morality requires adherence to unequivocal rules as indicative of a "taboo" mentality, which is inadequate because it fails to recognize the complexity of our moral world, in which we must often choose between conflicting values or principles. For Maguire, there are no straightforward rules that delineate the moral white from the moral black. Rather, one must be able to face the greys found in moral reality, in which simple solutions do not exist.

Maguire's claim echoes the beliefs of learning theorists J. Piaget, R. S. Peters, and L. Kohlberg. All of these theorists maintain that the moral development of children involves various stages, including an early one in which moral rules are construed as "given," absolute, and unalterable. Peters writes, "[Children] finally pass to the level of autonomy when they appreciate that rules are alterable, that they can be criticized and should be accepted on a basis of reciprocity and fairness. The emergence of rational reflections about rules . . . is the main feature of the final level of moral development."

The complexity of our moral life is a direct consequence of the fact that it embraces more than one principle or value, thus making conflict inevitable. One way to deal with such conflicts is to declare in advance that one value or principle will always take priority. This was essentially the strategy of those who dealt with the conflicting values of preserving life, minimizing suffering, and respecting patient autonomy, by insisting that all patients must always be treated aggressively. Physicians who adopted this strategy steadfastly refused to step onto the slippery slope. As we noted at the outset, however, most critical care providers find this position untenable precisely because it fails to acknowledge the conflict between values such as minimizing suffering and respecting patient autonomy.

Significantly, one steps onto the slope at the point that one acknowledges respect for competing values. Thus, those who are quite comfortable with withholding or withdrawing life-prolonging therapy for reasons of compassion or autonomy are already *on* the slope. Although those who are persuaded by Rachels' arguments may hold a position further down the slope than those who are not, it is simply a mistake to believe that his arguments must be resisted because they lure one *onto* the slope. It is crucial to realize, moreover, that those who would avoid this slope by always opting for aggressive treatment are, in fact, defining their position on competing slopes; competing values manifest themselves as "intersecting slopes." The fact that we also value respect for patient autonomy, for instance, gives rise to the "slope of medical paternalism"—that is, the range of possible views on when it is appropriate to disregard a patient's wishes. He who avoids stepping onto the "termination-of-treatment" slope by adhering to a policy of always treating aggressively, will do so without regard for the autonomy of the patient who cries "no more," thereby defining his position as rather unacceptably far down on the slope of paternalism. This, then, is the force of Maguire's claim that our moral world is too rich and complex to be handled adequately by a "taboo" mentality.

Maguire's rebuttal to the slope argument gains additional force from consideration of its role throughout history. Most major human advances in science, religion, or social order have occurred in spite of "slope" arguments akin to the one considered above. "If we permit research and experimentation in the areas of dissection of human cadavers/organ transplantation/genetic engineering/human reproduction, we open the door to a whole range of complicated moral considerations, which may be mishandled in a way that will lead to morally abhorrent practices." "If we allow people to develop methods of birth control which will tend to disassociate sex and reproduction, we invite moral decay and the destruction of the family." The same sort of argument has been made in closed societies against the questioning of established authorities. "While it's true that the authorities are sometimes mistaken, they serve the people well generally, and if dissenting opinions are allowed to be heard, there will be no place to draw a clear moral line between dissent and anarchy." From this argument some have concluded that people must not be allowed to stray onto the slippery slopes of free speech or religion or political dissent.

A final criticism points out that slope arguments can backfire. Berger and Berger, who favor a more conservative stand on abortion than that represented by *Wade v. Roe*, claim that the extreme "prolife" faction has actually used the "slope" argument in a way that has been counterproductive to their own goals. By insisting that no abortion is to be tolerated because all abortion is murder, "prolifers" are, in effect, claiming that abortion following rape or abortion to save the life of the mother is *as wrong as* abortion for convenience. But that, unfortunately, is logically equivalent to saying that abortion for convenience is *no worse* than abortion in these other circumstances. Having argued that there are no moral differences, they have actually enhanced popular belief in the slipperiness of the slope; this has, in turn, prompted some persons, who were initially sympathetic to abortion only following rape or to save the life of the mother, to believe that abortions under any other circumstances are equally acceptable.

We suggest that the slope argument is not merely faulty, but dangerous, if it leads us to believe we can avoid coming to grips with the moral complexities of situations in which the timing of death is the result of human decisions. We have suggested that some of the distinctions that currently figure in termination-of-treatment decisions do not serve us well; the principles that should guide such decisions are the same as those which prevail elsewhere—that is, respect for patient autonomy and the burden/benefit analysis which normally guides all other treatment decisions. These are the principles that can provide the surest moral footing on the slope. The simplicity of this framework should not belie the complexity that must be faced head-on when it is applied in actual critical care situations. We have tried to acknowledge some of the special problems associated with responsible decision making in this area, including those of patient competence, communication with patient and family, and, not least of all, legal ramifications.

Physicians must, of course, heed the legal reality of the situations in which termination-of-treatment decisions must be made and implemented. Unfortunately, the legal reality is sometimes even murkier than the moral one. In this connection, however, physicians should not view the courts as hopelessly conservative on these issues. Moreover, they should be aware of their own potential to influence those legal realities, for better or worse. We suggest that facing the moral issues as squarely as possible helps to ensure the best decisions in individual cases, and also optimizes the chances of clearer and saner legal precedents in the future. This observation is not naive and utopian. On January 7, 1985, the New Jersey Supreme Court authorized the withdrawal of feeding tubes from an 84-year-old incompetent patient who "had no cognitive abilities" and was terminally but not critically ill. Emphasizing the importance of previously expressed wishes, the court stated, "The right we are seeking to effectuate is a very personal right to control one's own life." In so doing, the court clearly rejected the distinctions between ordinary and extraordinary care, withholding and withdrawing treatment, and—explicitly—"the distinction that some have made between actively hastening death by terminating treatment and passively allowing a person to die of a disease." The spirit of the Court's decision echoes the findings of the Commission for the Study of Ethical Problems in Medicine and Biomedical and Behavioral Research report on *Deciding to Forego LifeSustaining Treatment.*

## CONCLUSIONS

We have argued that a number of distinctions traditionally considered morally significant in fact obscure the real basis on which rational decisions about prolonging life are made-namely, an analysis of burdens and benefits to be expected from any treatment option. Respect for patient autonomy requires that such analysis be made from the patient's perspective and, if he or she is competent, with his or her active participation. Since both assessment of competence and decision making in the absence of full competence fall largely to the physician, it is the physician who must orchestrate and implement treatment decisions. Such decisions are painful and complex enough without introducing irrelevancies.

# Chapter 10

# Ethical Issues in Critical Care Nursing

## INTRODUCTION

The ethical issues described by critical care nurses reflect all the dimensions of critical care settings described in earlier chapters. The setting, the rapidly changing technologies, and the evolving roles of nurses in critical care settings, all influence the ethical dilemmas that confront nurses, patients and their families, physicians, administrators, and many others who have prolonged contact in hospital settings.

Society is more and more bombarded with the consequences of contemporary medical treatment. The syndrome of multiple system failure and death from gradual deterioration and/or catastrophic events in a highly technological ICU (intensive care unit) setting is increasingly common. The social, financial, and human costs are immeasurable in such varied aspects of health care as organ procurement for transplants, fetal organ and tissue donation, and experimentation; treatment and privacy rights of patients with acquired immune deficiency syndrome (AIDS) and drug resistant tuberculosis (TB) versus risk to the public health, including the well-being of health care workers; reproductive issues such as contraception, abortion, surrogate parenting, extrauterine conception, and artificial insemination; and the rights of the aged in our society to health care. Issues of quality of life, death with dignity, right to die, and euthanasia emerge with increasing frequency in the treatment and care of terminally ill, dying, comatose, and brain dead individuals. Rapid changes in technology often seem to outpace the redesigning of social and legal structures and moral thought.

All these issues are influenced by problems and inequalities in society with regard to resource allocation and access to medical treatment. The economics of health care are tied to political and legislative processes and health policy. At the present time, many groups are underserved because of reduced or terminated services, especially the urban poor, women, particularly pregnant women, children, and minorities. This has consequences for institutional acute care. For example, a decrease in state funding for antepartal care reduces the number of outpatient services in urban areas. As a consequence, pregnant teenagers often receive no prenatal care. These women are already at high risk because of their age and frequently because of drug use or poor nutrition. Increasing numbers of these teenage mothers receive their first medical attention when they arrive in labor in an emergency room. In addition, many hospitals may turn a woman away if she has no proof of insurance. The risk is damage to mother and baby entailing a much higher financial burden to the individual, hospital, and society in terms of prematurity, neonatal ICU care, and long-term care of mentally or physically challenged children and adults than would be the cost of preventive prenatal care of the mother. Similarly, outpatient care for a child with asthma is much cheaper than emergency room care, hospitalization, or intensive care treatment of a child with respiratory distress. The consequences of these health care policies have changed the population of patients seen in hospital settings in the 1990s. Patients are older, younger, sicker, and in more distress prior to seeking treatment than in previous years.

Howard E. Freeman report the results of a 1986 study conducted by the Robert Wood Johnson Foundation about access to and use of health services between 1982 and 1986. The study reported that the gap in medical care between urban and rural residents had diminished and that most patients were satisfied with their physician and in-patient hospital care. Overall use of medical care had declined in terms of hospitalization and physician visits. Access to physician care for individuals who were poor, or uninsured had decreased, particularly for those in poor health. Hospitalization had also decreased for disadvantaged groups, but at a rate comparable to that of the general population. However, the uninsured patients received less hospital care than might be appropriate, given their higher rates of illness. Underuse of dental and medical services by key groups was reported; these groups included pregnant women in the first trimester, patients with diagnosed hypertension, and persons experiencing symptoms of significance such as bleeding (other than nosebleeds, menstrual periods, or bleeding caused by accident), shortness of breath after light exercise, loss of consciousness, chest pain, and unexplained weight loss of more than ten pounds. These findings confirm the growing problems of access of underserved groups to health care.

## DILEMMAS

Critical care nurses are directly involved with the sickest patients in the hospital system. They are also at the forefront of the ethical issues that have emerged as a consequence of treatment in critical care settings. These situations are complex, and the issues often are not clear. Simple logic and right or wrong judgment are insufficient as models of problem solving or analysis.

This chapter portrays the range of ethical dilemmas that critical care nurses have articulated as significant in their practice. The ethical dilemmas described by these nurses cover the following broad areas: issues related to death with dignity for dying patients, especially in circumstances associated with "do not resuscitate" (DNR) orders, realities surrounding organ transplant, and problems of resource allocation.

Ethics is defined as the body of moral principles or values governing good, evil, duty, and obligation in a particular culture or group. For example, infants are generally protected by social and legal codes, whereas in some cultures, infanticide is an acceptable method of population control. Morality in a given culture reflects the complex relationship between needs and rights. Many factors influence whether need fulfillment is a right, how persons are treated in a given society, and how the legal structure becomes formalized to reflect the social values. For the purposes of this discussion, ethics is understood in the Socratic tradition. Ethics is an attempt to formulate systematic responses to the question: What, all things considered, ought to be done in a given situation. Ethical inquiry in health care presumes a cognitive process of analytical decision making; a knowledge of legal, religious, and cultural constraints; and a consideration of role relationships, institutional constraints, and dependent, independent, and codependent functions of physicians and nurses.

Several writers in recent years have provided new insights into ethical issues in nursing practice. Anna Omery clarifies and defines values, moral reasoning, and ethics in nursing practice. Ketefian reviews and critiques measures and tools of moral reasoning and ethical practice in existing nursing research and concludes with very useful suggestions for future research. Elizabeth C. Reisman and Christine Grady address ethical principles related to nursing care of HIV-infected persons. These issues include, but are not limited to, the moral obligation to provide care and confidentiality and courage to face risks and impartiality to temper prejudice .

A five-step model of analysis for ethical decision making is presented by Martin Benjamin and Joy Curtis. First, they suggest, determine and obtain relevant factual information. Second, aim for clarity and draw relevant distinctions. Third, construct and evaluate arguments. Fourth, develop a systematic framework. Fifth, anticipate and respond to objections.

Increasingly, ethics committees exist in hospital settings to assist physicians, administrators, nurses, patients, and families with resolution of very complex ethical issues. In 1972, the Hospital Associations published "A Patient's Bill of Rights," delineating twelve areas of patient rights and hospital obligations, including the right to considerate, respectful, and continuous care; the right to information about diagnosis; the right to informed consent; the right to refuse treatment; the right to privacy; the right to reasonable treatment; and the right of access to the hospital record. Articulation of these rights and the formal establishment of ethics committees to assist decision making have helped to formalize the process of ethical decision making in medical care settings. The ethical dilemmas described by the critical care nurses reflect such a formal decision-making process. Rather, they reveal the perceptions of individuals caught up in the realities of the patient care situation. Making judgments and then deliberately acting on them is essential to the practice of nursing and medicine in hospitals. The decisions made affect the nurses and physicians, their patients, and the institutions and communities where they are located. Responsible decision making usually involves ethical choice but is rarely preceded by the complex and formal deliberation described by Benjamin and Curtis.

Ethical choice in nursing involves issues of accountability, responsibility, and legal definitions of nursing practice. Sigman has said, "Situations do not present themselves with labels attached.... The crux is in the labeling, or the decision...depends on how a situation is 'seen.'" Many factors will determine how a situation is "seen." The individual characters of nurses, their gender, race, financial status, and region of birth and personal development, and the nature of their socialization process into nursing education and practice are but a few of these factors. The roles that nurses fulfill in delivering patient care provide another window on the ways in which a situation is "seen."

Elsie and Bertram Bandman have identified the roles that nurses assume with patients that provide the basis for ethical choice.

The nurse-patient relationship fosters the two major roles of surrogate and advocate. The surrogate role implies complete trust, and the nurse is in a position of protecting the patient's most fundamental interests and rights, especially when the patient is helpless. The nurse becomes an agent for the patient in mediating between the patient's interests and the outside world. The nurse may be eyes, ears, arms, legs, and lungs for the patient, compensating for physiological or psychosocial deficits.

The role of advocate implies the protection of the patient's rights. The nurse may accomplish this through other roles such as health educator, technical expert, counselor, leader, or friend. Bandman and Bandman present three arguments rebutting the arguments against nurses as advocates. First, it is sometimes noted, nurses have no institutional protection when acting as patient advocate. Conflicts with physicians and others could cost the nurse his or her job. Bandman and Bandman respond that nurses may be projecting a future role. Patients' rights are in need of protection, and nurses are the logical persons to fulfill this role. Second, some physicians regard themselves as the primary patient advocate and resent intrusion by others. In response, Bandman and Bandman reply that all physicians are not always responsible and accountable. Further, as noted earliar, critical care nurses are increasingly liable for their own practice. Accountability for co-dependent practice is one aspect of this liability. Third, nurses may assume too many simultaneous roles to have the time, skill, and ability to serve as advocates. Others, for example lawyers, may be better trained for the advocacy role. The rebuttal to this argument is one of the predominant themes stated by critical care nurses. No other group has more continuous contact with patients and families than do nurses. Nurses are often the most familiar with patients' and families' ethical choices and are in a good position to protect those interests in critical care situations.

The professional organizations have formalized codes of ethics. The Nurses' Associations code for nurses published in 1976 and revised in 1985 gives eleven precepts addressing issues of patient privacy, respect for human dignity, competence, and a commitment to the public health. Of particular note is a reference to the role of advocate: "The nurse acts to safeguard the client and the public when health care and safety are affected by the incompetent, unethical, or illegal practice of any person" and "the nurse assumes responsibility and accountability for individual nursing judgement and actions".

Contemporary medical treatment has produced a changed set of circumstances surrounding death in the hospital setting. Several social trends and shifts have contributed to these changes. People are living longer and are surviving previously fatal diseases to die of something else. Individuals are, in increasing numbers, being treated and dying in hospitals rather than at home. Technology – notably, cardiopulmonary resuscitation (CPR) and equipment and procedures to perform the functions of the vital organs, or to replace the heart, lungs, kidneys, pancreas, liver, and bone marrow – has extended life and death beyond previously defined limits of medical intervention. These same trends have changed both the definition of death and the nature of the care that dying patients receive in hospitals. Both these issues will be explored later in this chapter.

Death was long regarded as a natural and inevitable outcome of illness, disaster, or longevity. Increasingly, as interventions became more successful, death was often postponed or held in abeyance. Since the development of cardiopulmonary resuscitation, a radical shift has occurred in the approach to death in the hospital setting and elsewhere. Surviving illness was once considered the rare occurrence. Death was far more common and regarded as the norm. Since the demonstrated effectiveness of CPR at restoring life, resuscitation is a requirement in hospital settings unless specific orders of "do not resuscitate" (DNR) are arranged for a particular patient. Challenging death has emerged as the norm. Criteria for determining candidates for resuscitation are not clear, although some texts attempt to state criteria such as "all others should be regarded as candidates for resuscitation, except those with known terminal illness and those who have been clinically dead for more than five minutes". In practice, all hospitalized individuals who die must have CPR initiated, unless a current DNR order has been written by the attending physician after documented consultation with patient, family, or guardian. The Joint Commission on Accreditation of Healthcare Organizations requires that all hospital personnel receive training and review of CPR techniques, at least annually.

The changes in intervention for death in hospitals have created great diversity in outcomes for patient prognosis. Successful resuscitation may result in complete recovery, initiation of artificial means of life support in a brain dead individual, or many stages in between. Unsuccessful resuscitation results in death, but a death surrounded by strangers, equipment, and chaos. As these patterns of treatment became universal in hospitals, they gave rise to many ethical issues, including appropriate levels of intervention and care for DNR patients with regard to diagnostic tests, surgery, administration of blood and antibiotics, and especially feeding and hydration. The dilemmas of achieving death with dignity, or a peaceful, comfortable death, were also exacerbated. Hospitals, as O'Mara has noted, are increasingly offering patients the opportunity and refining procedures for competent and ethical decision making. Further, various professional groups are attempting to establish codes of ethics and guidelines for intervention with regard to withdrawing or withholding food and fluids .

Nurses expressed a great deal of satisfaction about situations where patients were allowed to die with dignity when death was inevitable (as in brain death or multiple system failure) or appropriate (as in end-stage terminal illness). They expressed considerable frustration about those times when patients were not allowed to die with dignity, as when inappropriate resuscitation or extraordinary treatment was instituted or not withdrawn or when life-support care was continued beyond the patient's request. Communication seemed to be a key issue in these situations. Nurses facilitated communication between patients and families, patients and doctors, and families and doctors. As painful as the losses of dying could be for patients, families, and the medical team, the mechanical support of brain dead patients was worse, and was described as stressful and dehumanizing. Nurses were grateful when decisions were made and treatment plans, developed in conjunction with nursing, medicine, patient, and family, were clear. When technological possibilities dictated the care received, the treatment seemed to assume a life and momentum of its own. Participation in that process was described as devastating. Even in the presence of communication, language often failed. In the presence of hope for life, how can one explain the dehumanizing consequences of treatment.

Pate makes several succinct points. The nurse is a skilled member of a team and is obligated to be vocal. The dilemmas experienced by nurses in those situations are also felt by physicians. And the legal system has begun to reflect some of the social changes that have occurred as a result of rapid changes in life support technologies. The rights of patients to die with dignity when no hope exists of return to an acceptable quality of life are more and more protected. Another factor that has altered the entire medical and legal arena in the death with dignity issue is the evolution of the definition of death from the traditional cessation of heartbeat and breathing to the current one of brain death and/or documented persistent poor prognosis. The evolution of this definition was certainly influenced by both the use of the ventilator and the successful transplant of human organs and tissues.

Early respirators were used in the treatment of patients with polio and with near-drowning victims. After the 1950s, more refined ventilators were used successfully for temporary support after neurosurgery, cardiac surgery, myocardial infarction, and drug overdose. This technology has reduced mortality and is a useful tool. Ventilators are becoming increasingly common in both large urban hospitals and small rural ones. Since ventilators are as common in the long-term support of patients with multiple complications as they are in short-term crisis management, the problems associated with their use are more evident. The respirator can ventilate individuals who could not breathe on their own and who might also have loss of brain function. A person can "live" on the machine until death occurs from heart failure, infection, or some other cause. The dilemma of removing lifesupport technology is as problematic as initiating it. Because the technology exists, hospitals, nurses, and physicians are obligated to initiate lifesupportive, resuscitative efforts when a patient dies unless prior advisement with the patient and/or family and legal action have allowed a "do not resuscitate" order to be written. Hospitalized patients, even if terminally ill, are at the mercy of the technology, especially if a medical crisis or death occurs very quickly. Certainly long-term ventilator support has helped many persons to survive with good quality of life. The expense of such treatments and the dilemmas in decision making do not influence either the realities of initiating treatment or the likelihood of success or failure as outcome. The technology exists and is used.

"Death" ethicist Robert Veatch observes, "has always been inevitable. Where humans were once helpless observers in the presence of death, we are increasingly able to intervene in the process, using technological resources to direct or delay the inevitable." His observation seems to reflect humanity's struggle against death in the presence of ambivalence and fear. Paul Ramsey has described the role of contemporary health care personnel in this context: "The conviction that one should always choose life lies at the heart of the practice of medicine and nursing. Medical ethics must be pro-life in this context. This aspect of modern medicine was profoundly influenced by Judaism and Christianity" .The mandate to "choose life" appears absolute and definitive, yet no clarification is offered on the meaning of either quality of life or good and peaceful death. Society, in particular, denies death and conspires to keep it hidden from view. Modern funeral practices demonstrate this. The denial of death is focused in situations where death occurs in hospital settings, where technology is available to keep death at abeyance indefinitely. As G. H. Kieffer notes, "Death has been transformed from 'God's will' to a 'natural event' to an 'untimely event'".

The ventilator and artificial nutrition and hydration, either by a feeding tube into the stomach or bowel or by an intravenous line, have made extraordinary means of life support possible. Issues related to withdrawing or withholding food and fluids continue to be special problems for nurses, particularly in the care of severely handicapped newborns or patients with documented brain death. The issues are not completely identified or articulated, but efforts are underway by nurses, ethicists, legal advisors, consumers, and others to continue compassionate clarification of the human rights issues involved .

Concerns about artificial prolongation of the dying process, in many dying or critically ill patients or patients who are alert or who have made advance directives, have generated a debate about the issues involved in withdrawing or withholding artificial nutrition and hydration. L. S. Knox and M. E. Wurzbach (provide current literature and case review and sensitive discussions of these issues. The debate between humanitarian life extension and comfort versus selective withdrawal of nutrition and hydration will likely continue for some time. Certainly, critical care nurses are participants at the center of this debate. Similar concerns have emerged related to the withdrawal of mechanical ventilator support. Guidelines for terminal weaning and the ethical issues involved with goals for patient and family comfort are discussed in the recent literature .

The fourth edition of *Black's Law Dictionary*, published in 1968, reflected the traditional definition of death as "the cessation of life, the ceasing to exist, defined by physicians as a total stoppage of the circulation of the blood, and a cessation of the animal and vital functions consequent thereupon, such as respiration, pulsation, etc.". Machines that ventilate and circulate a body nourished by artificial means have rendered this definition meaningless. Technology created a semblance of life that must be distinguished from traditionally understood and valued styles of life and death. William May has articulated the problem well. "In the service of saving life," May writes, "heroic medicine can sometimes only assure that its final moments will be as miserable as possible. Humanity is tested in the way we behave toward death...and it is obscured and diminished when death is concealed from view,...when the dying are forced to make their exit anonymously, their ending unwitnessed, uncherished, and unrecorded except in the hospital files".

By the end of the 1970s, sophisticated intensive care units became commonplace in hospitals, and the possibilities of sustaining circulation and breathing, equated with "life," were a reality for almost all hospital patients. In the early 1980s, rapid pharmacological advances in immunosuppressant drug therapy precipitated a rapid emergence of organ transplant surgery. The capacity for successful organ transplant, and media attention to organ procurement and recipient issues, soon brought into focus the problems of traditional definitions of death, which were seen as obsolete. A donor organ had to be maintained by adequate circulation until transport to the recipient is initiated. If pronouncement of death in a donor was delayed until the heart or lungs stopped functioning, the life-saving transplant surgery could be jeopardized by deterioration of the donor organs. On the other hand, by the traditional definition of death, removal of vital organs before the heart and lungs failed constituted murder. These dilemmas illustrate the complexities involved and the need for a clear definition of death based on brain function.

Many cases were cited that documented the need for brain death legislation. A victim of a gunshot wound to the head provides an example. The "brain dead" patient was not pronounced dead by the physician until after the heart had stopped beating. The defendant, charged with murder, claimed that the patient did not die from a gunshot wound to the head (which had resulted in his brain death) but rather that the doctors had caused his death by removing his life support systems .

The Task Force on Death and Dying of the Institute of Society, Ethics and Life Sciences, in evaluating the Harvard criteria, voiced four areas of concern: the vagueness of the definition of death; the fear that the new criteria are primarily intended to facilitate transplants; mistrust of new powers vested in the attending physician; and fears that the new definition will lend itself to updating at an increasing risk to the dignity of the dying patient. Significantly, the Harvard criteria address only the definition of patient death, not when treatment should be withdrawn to allow the patient to die or when treatment should not be initiated.

The Harvard criteria for determining brain death or irreversible coma were soon validated in 1974 by the Royal College of the United Kingdom and in 1977 by further studies that established the credibility of the Harvard study findings. In the United States, individual states began, in 1971, to initiate brain death legislation. Since Kansas enacted the first statute in 1971, at least 25 states have passed brain death statutes with wide variance in language. The trend toward a uniform brain death statute was solidified by the independent adoption, in 1979, of a model statute, the

Uniform Brain Death Act, prepared by the American Bar Association, the American Medical Association and the National Conference of Commissioners on Uniform State Laws. This model statute, the Uniform Determination of Death Act, was endorsed by the Commission for the Study of Ethical Problems in Medicine and Biomedical and Behavioral Research, the Academy of Neurology, and the Electroencephalographic Society. Rather than stating explicit diagnostic criteria that might change with new technology, the statute supports the application of accepted medical standards for determining brain death. The statute reads, "An individual who has sustained either (1) irreversible cessation of circulatory and respiratory functions, or (2) irreversible cessation of all functions of the entire brain, including the brain stem, is dead. A determination of death must be made in accordance with acceptable medical standards". This act is adopted by most states at the present time.

Determination of brain death usually requires the independent assessment of another physician. The fifth edition of *Black's Law Dictionary* states the following definition of brain death: "A person shall be pronounced dead if it is determined by a physician that the person has suffered a total and irreversible cessation of brain function. There shall be independent confirmation of the death by another physician." The Harvard criteria provide the basis for determining brain death. By the time that the sixth edition of *Black's Law Dictionary* was published, the definition of brain death closely modeled the Uniform Determination of Death Act and the Harvard criteria: "Characteristics of brain death consist of: (1) unreceptivity and unresponsiveness to externally applied stimuli and internal needs; (2) no spontaneous movements or breathing; (3) no reflex activity; and (4) a flat electroencephalographic reading after 24 hour period of observation".

"Do not resuscitate" (DNR) orders, also referred to as "no code," are the source of much controversy for nurses and others caring for critically ill patients in hospitals. These patients may have a terminal illness, brain death, or a health status that is complex, complicated, and progressive in deterioration and hopelessness. A DNR order essentially means that cardiopulmonary resuscitative measures will be withheld in the event of acute cardiac or respiratory arrest. Given this definition, other forms of life-sustaining interventions such as antibiotics, feeding and hydration, and blood products can be and are administered to patients with DNR orders. In critical care units especially, where lifesaving technology is commonplace, decisions often must be made about which specific treatments should be initiated, withheld, or discontinued.

Lewandowski note that health professionals, families, and patients often disagree about the type and level of treatment to be provided to DNR patients. Attitudes range between two extremes, from the view that, except for CPR, all aggressive medical and nursing activities will be continued or initiated to the perspective that DNR patients should be allowed to die quietly and with dignity, a view that implies the withdrawal of life-sustaining medical intervention and the provision of only comfort measures. The researchers designed a study to examine the following three questions about DNR patients in a medical ICU. What levels of medical and nursing resources are consumed by DNR patients in the ICU. What is the impact of the DNR order and the withdrawal or initiation of life-saving and nursing interventions. Do DNR patients survive the ICU and hospital. A group of 506 patients admitted for one year to a medical ICU in an urban city were studied. Of these patients 71 were designated DNR during their hospital stay and none of the DNR orders were rescinded during the stay in the ICU. Of the DNR patients, 55 (77%) died in the ICU and another seven died on the medical ward after transfer from the ICU. Nine of the 71 patients lived and were discharged from the hospital. The mortality rate for the entire ICU population for the year was 17 percent.

The researchers examined resource consumption and nursing care requirements of both DNR and non-DNR patients in the ICU. Life-saving interventions, including ventilators, vasopressors, anti-arrhythmics, intravenous antibiotics, and pulmonary artery catheters, were continued on 73 percent of the patients who had them before the DNR order was written. A high percentage (91%) of ventilated patients remained on ventilators after being designated DNR. With the exception of ventilators, other treatments and diagnostic procedures (bronchoscopy, sigmoidoscopy, and abdominal ultrasound) were initiated on patients after DNR orders were written.

Nursing care requirements showed a similar trend. DNR patients required more nursing care than all other non-DNR patients, including those non-DNR patients who were seriously ill. A DNR designation did not alter the amount of nursing care required. DNR patients continued to have intense physical dependency needs and moderate to high social and emotional needs after the DNR order was written. Minimal rehabilitation and teaching were required both before and after the DNR order. The level of required observation decreased after the DNR order, although this reduced level was still assessed as being in the high to intense range.

The findings provide needed data both about the characteristics and treatment of DNR patients in a critical care setting and about the ambiguities involved in the meaning of the DNR order to patients, families, and health care personnel. The study reveals the following findings. It was common for DNR patients to occupy beds in an MICU (medical intensive care unit). Decisions about DNR designation and the appropriateness of varied levels of patient care were common issues in the critical care setting. DNR patients had very long ICU stays and consumed equal or greater medical and nursing resources than patients who were candidates for resuscitation. Patients who were DNR on the ward were transferred to the ICU. In fact, a DNR order was neither an indication that the physicians and nurses stopped caring for the patient nor a mandate for transfer out of the ICU.

Further, DNR patients continued to receive aggressive treatment. Although ventilation was not initiated after the DNR order, it was not withdrawn. Despite grave prognoses, physicians continued to treat DNR patients aggressively. Despite this level of intervention, the mortality rate remained very high. The issues of withdrawal of medical treatment and questions related to the most appropriate care for DNR patients remain largely unaddressed. Is an ICU the appropriate place for nurses to best meet the DNR patient's physical, psychological, and social needs. The researchers note the need for further studies to determine appropriate treatment and care of DNR patients. Continuation of aggressive medical treatment in a patient for whom resuscitation would mean a postponement of death wastes scarce ICU resources and causes undue patient suffering and crippling financial burdens for patients, families, and society. Finally, the researchers advise that future research be focused on the quality of life of DNR patients who survive hospitalization to determine the moral implications of treatment of DNR patients in the hospital setting.

Tittle, Moody, and Becker studied DNR and nonDNR patients in order to identify which variables are the best predictors of a DNR classification so that a model could be developed to predict the level of nursing care required by DNR patients in the ICU. One model identified the best predictor as the origin of admission and the severity of illness on the admission day. A second model identified the best predictor as the number of days spent in the ICU prior to the DNR order, the average daily resource allocation points after the DNR order, and the severity of illness scores on the day the DNR order was designated.

Jezewski studied self-reporting of 22 critical care nurses with at least one year of experience in a critical care unit to investigate the process of consenting to "do not resuscitate" status. A theoretical model was developed that considered issues of timing, the meaning of DNR to family members, areas of conflict, and the role of the nurse, including ongoing support of the patient and family.

These studies illustrate the ambiguities involved in treating very ill patients in critical care settings. Nurses are present continuously with these patients and their families during the duration of their ICU and hospital stays. The range of stresses, satisfactions, and frustrations that nurses experience in caring for patients for whom they perceive ethical dimensions of care are well known.

Pat Dalton addresses issues of language and informed consent. Patients can't really know what the consequences of treatment may involve if things do not go well. Dalton describes the impact on the nursing staff of providing that care:

I don't think we inform people enough. And I don't think that our socalled "informed consent" is really informed. They don't realize what they're going to be put through. But we go round and round all the time. We've got one surgeon that does open hearts on some of these patients that are high risks. He did a case — it's been a couple of months ago, but it was on a — he was a 54-year-old man...had been turned down at the Cleveland Clinic and the Mayo Clinic five years ago because he was such a poor risk. He had such bad heart disease. And this particular surgeon decided he was going to do him. He ended up in surgery a long, long time. He had a hard time getting him off bypass, and they were going to put a left ventricular assist device in him and all this kind of stuff. They finally got him off. The surgeon was there waiting for the patient to roll around, and I asked him, "Why did you do it." This particular doctor, he's only a couple of years older than me and I know he gets upset when his patients do badly and he gets real depressed when they die and it's a drain on him. But he said, "This man wanted it. He knew that if he didn't have it he was going to die and he wanted to take the chance." He said, "I had to do it." And this man did fine. Yet then we get another patient, the same surgeon did her. It was a young woman. She was about 40. But she looked about 30, I couldn't believe it. She was a real nice lady. She had no risk factors, but had a right ventricular AMI [acute myocardial infarction] all of a sudden. She wasn't a smoker and had no risk factors at all. She looked like a good risk for surgery. And he did her, and she died that night. So you never know, and I guess even though we say, "Why are we doing this to all these people." If it's their choice, who are we to say, "No, we're not going to do it." But then again, these people have got to know what can happen to them. Physicians always say, I don't know how many times I've heard it, "Well, everything that's wrong with them can be reversed." Well, that's fine, but if somebody's in respiratory failure, is in cardiac failure, is in renal failure, or liver failure, and is comatose – sure, each one of them may be reversible, but don't tell me that you know that person's going to get up and walk out. You just don't see that. We had a trauma. A young girl. I know she was young, but had 40 units of blood in like a three hour period. And you know right away that person's lungs are gone. They might as well forget that. Yet in the three-day period after that she must have gotten a hundred and more units of blood. And they tried to dialyze her and they did all that stuff. And she still died. They could have stopped days before and saved the family from any false hope that maybe she can get better, let alone from the expense people are being put through.

It's real frustrating when you see this. There's all this thing with informed consent with these open hearts. The physicians now are documenting in their progress notes, "The surgery was explained and the risk was explained for mortality, for bleeding, for stroke, was all written out for the patient with percentages." Nobody will ever convince me that these families and these patients realize that this risk for stroke could mean you're going to end up a vegetable for the rest of your life or on a ventilator for the rest of your life. They don't know what it means to be on a ventilator for the rest of your life. It's one thing if they tell you your risk of dying in surgery is 10 percent. Fine, if I'm going to die in surgery I'm going to die there, but they don't realize what it means to sit on that ventilator for the rest of your life. They don't realize what it means. They're told there's a one percent chance of infection. Big deal. People get infections all the time. They don't realize the sternum can get infected and it comes open and you can see their heart beating and we're putting dressings on top of the heart. They don't realize what that means, you know. And we keep doing it to these people. That's what is real frustrating to me. And we're seeing it more and more now too.

Appropriate medical and nursing care requirements of terminally ill or hopelessly ill patients in the ICU setting remain uncertain and debatable due to many factors. The Lewandowski study deals primarily with appropriate levels of care for patients already designated DNR. The data reveal many other aspects of the ethical dimension of caring for patients who are brain dead or hopelessly ill.

First, nurses discussed the pain, stresses, and frustrations of dealing continuously with patients who are brain dead or hopelessly ill, when the family or physician, because of legal entanglement or philosophy, persist in denial or indecision about designating a patient DNR. Because nurses are there so consistently, they must deal with the consequences of decisions made by others as well as the outcomes of decisions others will not make. Nurses experience a great deal of conflict, for several reasons, if they perceive that decisions are not in the patient's best interest. Nurses are present continuously and implement the specifics of care. Family members often approach the nurses, rather than the physicians, for rationale or explanations about care the physicians have not offered. Decisions made or not made by physicians or family – for example, decisions to withdraw treatment or to refuse to treat or to treat aggressively in persons in older age groups – may conflict with the nurses' value system, beliefs, or professional judgment.

Second, nurses described the difficulties associated with the meaning of language and communication in the critical care setting. Nurses were caught in a situation of crisis when physicians, because of fear of lawsuits, lied to family members about brain death in children or when physicians were unable to come to a decision about when to stop aggressive treatment, designate a patient DNR, and allow the patient to die with dignity. Nurses, especially nurse managers, were often effective in these situations in helping to establish policies to facilitate decision making about brain death or "no code" procedures. Nurses also facilitated or initiated discussion with physicians about stopping treatment.

Issues of language also present complex dilemmas for nurses in critical care settings. The language of "informed consent" is difficult, even for the most conscientious physician. Patients must be presented with a range of risks and benefits by the physician offering a particular treatment. As treatment options have become more complex and invasive, the consequences of long-term management of complications in patients who do not do well become awesome. Nurses described the conflicts inherent in caring for persons who, in hope of a good outcome, chose a procedure, but did not do well.

The conflicts in this scenario are major components of the realities of contemporary critical care practice for patients, families, physicians, and nurses.

Patients hope for positive outcomes, and this hope may influence recovery. Success and failure are not yet predictable. Patients do well who should not, and others die who seem to be excellent risks. Families and patients, in crisis, often may not "hear" the risks as they are explained. Physicians, with varying communicative skills, may deny the possibilities of failure so much that they cannot express them. And even if the risks are explained, language may be inadequate to express the reality. People cannot really know what it is like to live on a ventilator for the rest of one's life. Similarly, infections rarely can be interpreted as seeing one's open chest or abdomen.

The third outcome of data deals with the conflicts and stresses associated with caring for DNR patients. "DNR" may be interpreted as "no care" by nurses, physicians, family, or nursing administration, although the DNR patient is often in ICU on a ventilator. Nurse staffing may often be reduced by management and actual levels of care may be reduced by nurses themselves, although the DNR patient's care requirements are, as Lewandowski notes, often equal to that of acutely ill patients. Nurses often experienced conflict over being caught between family members and physicians regarding degrees of aggressiveness in care, the absence of clear and honest communication, and implementing specifics of care they believed were causing pain or were not in the patient's best interest.

Nurses develop strategies for coping with these dilemmas themselves and also for helping patients and families survive the pain. Nurses need to have hope in patient situations, if not for patient survival or quality of life, at least for clear communication and decision making and death with dignity. Even when patient situations are hopeless and dehumanizing, nurses are there, continuously, with patients and their families. Nurses are there, caring for the patient, whatever the reality. Nurses are there in a personal way for dying patients when they were alone. They support family members to assist them in accepting the reality that they made the best decision possible at the time under the circumstances. Nurses implement policies that protect patients' rights when decisions about DNR status have not been made. Nurses facilitate communication between physicians and families and coordinate all hospital services dealing with the patients' care.

Nurses are there and are willing to be available to dying patients. They sense when patients are tired and ready to die. They also may support physicians as they work through their own grief in the process of letting someone die. Hardeman observes, "You stay there till it is over." Helping someone to die is painful, but almost a gift. The dehumanization of the artificial life support is far worse.

The ethical dilemmas experienced by nurses seem related to rapid changes in medical technology that often outpace structural and human adaptation and to the roles that nurses assume with patients, families, and physicians in critical care settings. Nurses are the single most persistent factor in the care of critical care patients. This presence involves nurses in the ambiguities of care of patients with multi-system failure and in care of patients where right to die, DNR, and quality of life are significant issues. Nurses are also involved in the types and levels of treatment that DNR may mean in patient care.

The ethical dilemmas created when extraordinary treatment was initiated or continued inappropriately and patients were not allowed to die with dignity caused much stress and conflict for the critical care nurses. The major sources of stress seem related to the following factors. Nurses are at the bedside continuously and are carrying out the procedures that may be perceived by patients and by the nurses themselves as cruelty and torture. Indecision by others, especially family or physicians, may prolong this period of dehumanization. Physicians and nursing administrators may be more oriented toward "cure." Although care for DNR patients remains demanding and time-consuming, medical support in patient management and nurse staffing in units with DNR patients may actually be diminished. Especially in cases where decisions are not made, nurses may be the persons required to initiate resuscitative efforts on hopelessly ill patients if they die before DNR decisions are made.

The roles that the critical care nurses assumed to cope with these ethical dilemmas were essentially the same roles that they assumed in other patient care situations. Significantly, as patient care becomes more complex, nurses continue to be involved in both independent and interdependent ways. Nurses reported involvement in initiating policy changes in hospitals related to brain death legislation. Other nurses described experiences of carrying out the actual care of patients, who, after court orders were obtained, were made comfortable and removed from lifesupport systems.

Nurses spoke of other roles that they used in caring for patients caught in these ethical dilemmas. These roles and behaviors include advocacy; management and coordination of the total patient care situation; communication with patient, family, physicians, and others, especially interpretation of the medical environment for the patient and family; shared intimacy with patients and an ability and willingness to use that for the patient's well-being; assessment of subtle changes in patient status and identification of trends; physical presence with patients who are dying, especially those who are dying alone; physical care and comfort measures; and support of patients, families, and physicians in the realities of painful decision making. Nurses voiced repeatedly that their motivation for and major satisfaction with nursing rests in making a difference in the lives of patients in crises. That nurses report having been able to do this so persistently, in such diverse settings, despite rapid change, stresses, and a host of other inhibiting factors, seems to make this a pivotal issue for consideration as society deals with the problems of maintaining adequate nursing care.

## Chapter 11

# Issues in Critical Care Nursing

## INTRODUCTION

Nurses as individuals and nursing as a discipline are obscure in written histories. Nursing is often viewed in the shadow of the history of medicine, and even when the story of nursing is told, problems exist in finding appropriate primary source materials. While the details of nursing education and professional organization are well documented, the story of the development of actual clinical practice is almost non-existent. Further, written histories of nursing almost always demonstrate region, class, and sex bias; most written histories represent the activities of middle- and upper-class women. The development, since the 1960s, of clinical specialization has received even less attention by scholars.

The development of critical care nursing is tied to developments in medical specialization after World War II and the increasing use of highly complex technology in the hospital care of patients. The trend to locate very ill and dependent patients with highly skilled nurses began with the recovery room experience in the 1940s and 1950s.

Improved techniques in cardiac surgery and developments in equipment for monitoring and manipulating cardiac status at the bedside accelerated this trend. The surgical and medical intensive care units (ICU) appeared in the 1950s and the coronary care units (CCU) in the 1960s. By the late 1960s, ICUs and CCUs were common in hospitals of all types and sizes. Community hospitals would commonly have a large combined medical-surgical ICU and a separate CCU, while university teaching hospitals might have multiple ICUs representing medical and surgical specialties such as heart surgery, pulmonary, organ transplant, burn care, and the like. Patients in the 1990s might be admitted to an ICU for an acute illness like a heart attack; for short-term management after specialized surgery such as removal of a brain tumor; or for long-term management of complications of either, such as respiratory support on a ventilator after a postoperative stroke or pneumonia.

Political, economic, and social realities have changed the health care establishment and the populations requiring care. Patients are older and sicker at every age when they arrive for treatment at the largely "illnessoriented" and "crisis-oriented" medical system. Increasing numbers of individuals are denied access to medical treatment, and these factors have supported the call for reform of the health care system. The highly invasive medical and surgical interventions available in medical care require a complex technology, very specialized and skilled medical and nursing support, and multiple ancillary personnel and support structures. While these interventions result in effective treatment and improved longevity for many, the outcomes for persons who do not do well are severe. These individuals may spend their last days in impersonal environments, on lifesupport equipment, among strangers. Further, procedures and decision making regarding the use or discontinuance of extraordinary life support technologies are unclear and incremental, respectively.

## DIFFERENT SCENARIOS

These acute care and life-support scenarios occur daily in critical care units. Nursing is the persistent factor in the development and operation of the critical care unit. Specialization in nursing followed that of medicine. At the same time many technical support occupations emerged to manage the developments in medical technology. Nursing embraced the technology, acquired the skills, and assumed the task of teaching new nurses critical care content. The nurse, the patient, and the equipment "became" the critical care unit. Nursing incorporated these skills into traditional roles. While other groups concentrated on one system or focus – such as respiratory care or mobility – the nurse assumed total responsibility for round-the-clock care of the patient and all equipment that appeared at the bedside, although the ICUs might be distinguished by medical or surgical specialty.

The direct care role of the nurse has become very complex and sophisticated. The nurse maintains the equipment, generates vast amount of data, and makes decisions about patient care based on assessment of the data and the patient's total physical and emotional status. Frequently, the nurse initiates, modifies, or terminates treatment based on those assessments. Physicians and others depend on the nurse to call them to the patient's bedside when they are needed. In addition, the nurse "extends" the physiological or psychological functions of person's unable to care for themselves due to illness or injury. For example, the nurse will turn paralyzed patients and facilitate bowel, bladder, and skin integrity and will manage the airway and manipulate oxygenation in patients on respirators, who are unable to breathe for themselves.

The ICU environment also has become very complex. Illnesses that place patients in ICUs are crises, often sudden, painful, and debilitating in their impact on patient and family. The nurse becomes the primary figure and contact person for family members. The ICU environment and patient care have become increasingly risky as a result of the use of toxic or dangerous products such as plastics, chemicals, drugs, chemotherapeutic agents and radiation, and the introduction of highly contagious and incurable diseases such as hepatitis B, non-A non-B (C) hepatitis, and Acquired Immune Deficiency Syndrome. Infectious and toxic agents of particular concern to pregnant women and to men and women concerned with genetic damage to themselves such as cytomeglian virus (CMV), radiation, and toxic chemotherapeutics are increasingly present in hospitals.

The ICU environment, the high technological and emotional demands of patient care, and the organizational styles of management in some hospitals have been found to be very stressful, often contributing to burnout in nurses. The impact of this environment has received the attention of Spicer and Robinson, who propose a conceptual model of the critical care work environment. A nursing shortage has been persistent in hospitals since soon after World War II, but has assumed crisis proportions in the 1990s. Ninety-seven percent of nurses are employed, and even though the actual number of nurses has shown a steady increase for the past twenty years, the increase has not kept pace with the demand. This shortage is thought to be due to an increasing demand for nurses and a diminishing supply. At the same time that increasing numbers of highly skilled nurses are needed, fewer women are attracted to nursing and nurses in the field are leaving for other careers. L. H. Aiken, in considering the future of hospital nursing, proposes new roles or career tracks in hospital nursing, designed to parallel the organization of medical care in hospitals. Aiken cautions that, although hospitals must be financially stable to survive, "Overidentification with the concerns of management and preoccupation with the day-to-day operation of the institution divert nurses' time, attention, and perhaps even loyalties away from patients and away from the clinical challenges and common interests they share with physicians".

Altruism and caretaking have been consistent themes throughout the history of nursing. The economics of nursing as a predominantly female occupation, the current nursing shortage, and the value of caring ascribed by society and by nurses themselves are some of the issues related to the altruism of nursing that scholars have not sufficiently explored. The combination of altruism and competence peculiar to critical care nursing remains unexplored in a systematic way. As Vreeland and Ellis have noted, warmth and sympathy are expected from ICU nurses together with objectivity and assertiveness. This conflicting demand contributes to the stress experienced by nurses in ICU settings.

The nurse became the most persistent treatment figure in the critical care unit because of skill, competence in judgment, and round-the-clock presence. The growth in technology, medical specialization, and knowledge focused the need to place the nurse with the patient in the critical care unit. The need to locate the nurse with the patient seems to be the guiding force behind this planning, rather than the need to manage the equipment. In fact, the early units in the 1950s opened without special monitoring equipment. The nurse was the monitor, and the private duty model seemed the appropriate one to illustrate this nurse-patient relationship. As technology changed continuously and very rapidly, the nurse added the new skills to the traditional caretaking roles that had been the domain of nursing. The nurse became the critical care unit. Vast amounts of data were generated, and again the nurse incorporated additional skills into the scope of practice. In fact, nurses had always made clinical judgments about patient care. But critical care increased the pace and the complexity of these judgments and subsequent acts.

Nurses perceived technology with ambivalence, appreciating the successful outcomes for patients but experiencing great conflict with its use. Technology was expensive and time-consuming and generated a great deal of data that often was not used appropriately. Medicine and nursing at times became overreliant on technology at the expense of the manual physical assessment skills of palpitation, auscultation, observation, and percussion. Roles became unclear, and questions became increasingly common about the appropriate uses of technology. The existence of technology, rather than individual patient need, often seemed to dictate its use. Nurses expressed frustration in those situations since the technologies were often invasive and painful for patients, and often the nurse was the person implementing the treatments. Technology compressed the time available to teach patients in even a minimal way about their illness. As technology became more pervasive, the human dimension of care seemed compressed and compromised.

The technology at the bedside – monitors, drug titrations, drains, infusions, everything attached to the patient – became the on-going responsibility of the nurse. The caring, skill, and continuous presence of the nurse were accompanied by a new aggressiveness.

*The commitment of critical care nurses to patients and to nursing practice is passionate and personal. They believe that they make a difference to patients through competence, caring, coordination and management of the clinical environment, and advocacy.*

The critical care nurses expressed great commitment about self, nursing, and caretaking. Many described nursing as a vocation. Nurses believed that they made a difference in the lives of others in crisis through competence in the care delivered, management of the patient's clinical situation, and the relationship they established with patients and their families. Even nurses who were neutral about expressing a vocational commitment were heavily invested in patients, nursing, or the clinical situation. None of the nurses were indifferent, negative, or impersonal about patient care or nursing.

Nurses valued their patient contact even as the skill level increased. The nurse-patient interaction was the greatest source of motivation and satisfaction that nurses expressed. Hence, those same situations were frustrating when patients were caught in crises of indecision about the uses of technology, especially extraordinary treatment. Since nurses were constantly present with patients, patients and often their families confided secrets to nurses, and frequently the nurse would serve as mediator between patients and their physicians or their own family members. Nurses felt that they were a humanizing link for patients and families in the impersonal hospital environment. For example, the terms "instant intimacy," "taking care of patients," and "making a difference" were expressions used often to describe the kinds of communication, advocacy, and physical and emotional bond nurses experienced with patients. This was accomplished through teaching, interpreting the medical or hospital system, manipulating details of the environment to meet a goal, and performing multiple tasks simultaneously to "make the hospital system work for patients."

Performing many tasks at one time involved providing "hands-on" physical care, communicating with and coordinating many individuals and groups, and managing physiological imbalances in unstable patients. Nurses recognize subtle changes and patterns, and intervene before a crisis event occurs. Physicians are dependent on nurses for this function. Most often, the physician would not be aware of a patient problem unless alerted by a nurse. Nurses report special satisfactions and skill in caring for dying patients and for patients in pain. Nurses use touch, relaxation, and creative presence in these situations.

## ROLE FUNCTIONING

The satisfactions of intimacy with patients and the challenges of clinical care occur at a cost. Nurses indicated that many stresses exist in these environments. These stresses include: feeling responsible and in fact being expected to meet the totality of a person's needs when the nurse has limited authority for autonomous decision making; the care itself (for example, being constantly involved with dying patients); the constraints of the job (for example, lack of administrative support, inflexible hours, heavy demands, perceived low self-esteem, and inadequate staffing patterns in the ICUs); and the rapidly changing and complex technology, especially if indecision regarding its use results in prolonged patient suffering.

These increased levels of role functioning with patients, physicians, and others resulted in increased status and self-esteem for some nurses. Others expressed almost a schizophrenic ambivalence about nursing, hospitals, and medicine because of stress and the lack of clarity in their roles.

Nurses expressed great satisfaction when patients were allowed to die with some element of humanity and dignity, if death was inevitable. As painful as dying could be, artificial life support was worse, especially for nurses, because they provide the care that they may perceive as "torture" and "dehumanizing." Nurses felt so personally involved with patients that participation in such care was seen as a violation of patient wishes and a betrayal of trust. Conflicts in decision making among patients, families, and physicians were the major sources of stress in these situations. Nurses perceived that they often facilitated decision making and communication at these difficult times. They often recognized when patients were tired and helped communicate this to families or physicians. They also reported that they provided support to physicians when "it was time to quit." The dilemmas seem to emerge from the technological capacity to extend life. One nurse said, "The ability to do has outstripped the ability to decide when doing is appropriate."

The issues involved with "do not resuscitate"(DNR) were the most frequently cited dilemmas related to death with dignity. The stresses nurses experienced before DNR decisions were made resulted from the uncertain ties about intervention. The nurse would be the person to initiate life support on a person for whom she perceived no hope of return to quality of life, if DNR decisions were not made before death. After the DNR decision was made, the stresses related to the ambiguities about appropriate levels of medical and nursing care. On the one hand, DNR care might be interpreted as all intervention except resuscitation. Often nurse staffing was reduced in ICUs if DNR patients were present. Some nurses reported that nurses themselves interpreted DNR to mean little or no nursing care.

This issue of appropriate levels of care portrays an underlying theme that has been persistent in the history of ICUs – who needs ICU care. Critical care has at times been interpreted as justified for those individuals who will recover to some quality of life. From this perspective, terminally ill patients do not require a critical care bed. These attitudes and values have been variable and influenced by the resources available – such as the number of ICU beds available or the level of financial reimbursement for services. Rapid increases in technology, the increased availability of ICU beds, and the highly invasive procedures performed in the 1990s have created a situation where many ICU beds are filled with patients suffering from the end-stage consequences of disease and/or treatment. These realities exist along with the differing views of who deserves ICU care. These issues have not been addressed, except in an economic sense. Hospitalization, treatment, and ICU care are generally available for those who can pay.

The incongruities involved in issues related to language, informed consent, and the realities of care of patients dying from the consequences of disease or failed treatment represented other ethical dilemmas for critical care nurses. Hope versus risk were very real, and language was inadequate to express the realities of "living the rest of your life on a ventilator" or "seeing your heart beating in your open, infected chest cavity." Nurses experienced these conflicts because of their commitment to patients and because they were there so constantly providing the care.

Nurses described the realities of caring for patients who, at their request, were removed from life-support equipment and allowed to die peacefully. In these situations, nurses were involved in facilitating decision making and legal processes and providing the drugs and emotional and physical support at the time of death. One nurse said, "You stay till it's over."

This persistence in caring and remaining at the bedside does have limits. Nurses reported a high degree of stress and burnout in ICU settings. Very little was found in the literature or heard in the interviews about successful measures to reduce nurse burnout. The issue is complex and likely related to the status and self-perception of women, the status and realities of nursing in hospitals, and the value of caring.

Nurses feel ambivalence and conflict about the necessary and difficult relationship between nursing and both medicine and the hospital as an organization.

As care became complex, nurses and physicians in critical care settings worked persistently and closely together. Both groups had specialized skills and communicated in complex ways. Ambiguities often existed in roles, relationships, male-female interaction, and distinctions of power and influence. Critical care nurses and physicians shared expertise and knowledge in various medical and surgical specialties that excluded other nurses and physicians. Nurses assumed many roles that had been within the traditional domain of medicine – physical assessment, determining drug dosage and titration based on physiological criteria, initiating or withdrawing invasive lines or tubes. This close association resulted in expert care for patients with particular problems, for example renal failure or heart transplant.

However, the priorities, values, and status of the two groups are often at variance. The physician retains the power of ultimate, formal decision making with regard to patient care. Nurses and some physicians (for example, specialists in anesthesia, radiology, and pulmonary medicine) are hospital employees and, along with consulting physicians, physical therapists and nurses are in a position to recommend or use formal and informal methods to influence care.

Nurses described several examples of frustration in dealing with physicians. These included indecision about designating a patient DNR; being deceptive with patients, families, or nurses; refusing to come and see critically ill patients when called by a nurse; and continuing painful treatment on patients against their wills, when death is inevitable, either because of research goals or physician denial. Nurses also reported instances of excellent rapport with physicians where they felt mutual respect for skill and support in coping with the shared losses in critical care. The relationship between nursing and medicine deserves further study relative to the changing status of medicine in society, the crisis of hospital care related to the nursing shortage, the support systems available to both medicine and nursing, and the changes in health care brought about by the increased focus on prevention and health promotion, a more informed consumer and managed care and prospective payment systems.

The conflicts in nursing practice related to the nurse as hospital employee represent an area that has received little attention by scholars. The personal commitment and nursing practice philosophy of the individual critical care nurse are directly influenced by how effectively a particular hospital is managed. Nurses described the stress and frustrations when nurse staffing was inadequate to provide minimally safe care to patients, when in fact hospitals could close beds to maintain adequate nurse-patient ratios or increase nurse-staff ratios. When these staffing patterns became rather frequent events, nurses exercised the only control they had. They left that hospital for another job or they left nursing for another career. Staffing patterns, more than any other, were described as the one final stressor that, added to the many others, made nurses consider leaving the setting or the occupation.

Nurses consistently expressed that "making a difference to patients" was their primary motivation for nursing. These same values were expressed by the nurses currently in administrative positions in hospitals. Yet practicing nurses experienced impotence and felt that they were treated with indifference by administrators. Nurses felt that they were valued less as individuals and more as anonymous pawns. "A nurse is a nurse is a nurse. I'm not valued as an individual or as a person of value." It is important to remember that the nurses voicing these feelings are the ones still in the settings providing the care. Nursing and hospital administrators would do well to examine the conflict between professional nursing practice and employment in the bureaucratic organization of the hospital. The private duty model, where patients and nurses contracted for service, exists in nursing history as a focus for study. Certainly, patients require adequate nursing care in hospitals, and that care must be provided efficiently. This issue may be one component of the problem with the medical care system.

Voices of critical care nurses reflect the values of the individual and the culture at any point in time. These examples reflect attitudes and values of individuals, educational institutions, and hospitals at particular points in time in particular places.

Several examples of racial prejudice and the ways in which prejudice influenced the ranges of medical options offered and the quality of care provided were discussed. Two nurses described care provided to siblings in crisis with sickle cell anemia. Both described indifferent medical care and spoke of nursing care that consistently underestimated pain. These nurses learned about comfort measures caring for these siblings at home, and both nurses reported that these experiences were a motivation for nursing as a career.

A nurse described the cultural tradition in the community to reject the offer of "do not resuscitate" designation for patients who have no hope of recovery. She attributed this reluctance to mistrust of the medical system.

She also noted the characteristic faith in God in the community: "Man does all that he can and God will take care."

A nurse reported that in hospitals she had witnessed that fewer aggressive medical options had been offered to patients who were poor. She felt that the philosophy of the attending physician and the degree of aggressiveness of family members were the primary determinants.

This view of the experiences of the practicing critical care nurse documented the personal characteristics and commitments of nurses to patients and nursing, the progression of a largely female occupational group, and the values of the larger society as health care has become complex, highly technical, and invasive. The values experienced in this book represent those of committed, motivated nurses who are still in practice settings. The realities of mediocrity, indifference, and burnout in nurses and physicians in critical care deserve the attention of scholars. This study portrays some of the diverse characteristics of critical care settings.

Nurses were the persistent human factor in the critical care settings described. They consistently expressed a commitment to patients and demonstrated the ability to assume highly complex and sophisticated patient care skills. The settings where critical care is practiced and the nature of patient care itself are stressful. These stresses and existing conflicts between the professional goals of nursing and the economic realities of the hospital as employer may further increase a serious shortage of nurses internationally. While care has become increasingly complex, hospitals are "downsizing" and cutting nursing positions, both at the bedside and in support roles. Many nurses are reflecting on the personal costs of providing that care with fewer nurses in settings that are increasingly ambivalent to some of the aims of nursing.

Further, caring has been a traditionally feminine attribute. The ways in which nurses and nursing, hospitals, and the larger society value and define that caring may determine the existence or demise of nursing in the future. Patients in contemporary critical care settings are vulnerable and require nursing care. These settings will become even more complex. Nursing has not sufficiently defined and protected its scope of practice so that the critical elements of nursing care are assured. This leaves nursing and patients vulnerable to the economic priorities of for-profit groups.

Patient care and a willingness to combine that with performance of expert skills. The goals of nursing seem congruent with the trends in health care that reflect consumer participation, prevention, health promotion, and a demand for institutional accountability. Nurses expressed commitment to such goals. The interpersonal contract between nurse and patient would seem the likely model for professional practice expressed by the nurses. Critical care nursing represents a model of professional and institutional practice that is unique at the present time. Critical care nursing may be able to translate that particular combination of competence and caring into formal power in the hospital setting for the good of nursing and for the humane and ethical care of patients.

# Index

## I



## L



## M



## N



## O



## R



## S



## T



## U